D1756930

The Metabolic Reset

Unlock the Secrets to Revitalizing Your Slow
Metabolism

David Alexander

Bohemian Publishing Group LLC

Contents

Introduction

Welcome to a pivotal turn in your journey toward health and vitality. You're about to embark on a transformative path that's not just about shedding pounds but fundamentally resetting the way your body processes energy. This book, which unfolds over the following chapters, isn't just another diet guide—it's a blueprint to revitalize your metabolism and, by extension, your life.

Perhaps you've noticed changes in your body, a certain sluggishness that wasn't there before, or maybe you're finding it harder to lose weight despite trying all the known tricks in the book. It can be disheartening, no doubt, but here's some encouraging news: what you're experiencing isn't a life sentence. Your metabolism isn't fixed; it's programmable. And you're holding the code.

Understanding metabolism is our first port of call. It's a term tossed around often, usually linked to weight and energy, but do you know what it truly entails? It's the complex biochemical process where your body converts what you eat and drink into the energy it's so dependent on—running the gamut of functions from breathing to circulating blood to repairing cells.

Now, let's address a pressing concern. Many of you may believe metabolism is dictated solely by things out of your control—age, sex, or genetics, for instance—but that's only part of the picture. While these factors do play a role, lifestyle and environmental elements hold significant sway over your metabolic rate. This revelation alone is empowering; it means there's room for change, and it's within your grasp.

Of course, we must also bust some persistent myths about metabolism. Misinformation abounds, and we'll dismantle these fallacies piece by piece, setting the stage for the truths that empower us.

As you continue through this journey, you may recognize symptoms of a slow metabolism. It's important to understand how this state of being can impact both body and mind—not to frighten you, but to arm you with awareness. And when exactly should you seek professional medical advice? We'll get there.

The crux of this book—metabolic reset—is an endeavor grounded in science, not whimsy. Here, hormones are central characters, with insulin, glucagon, and thyroid hormones playing lead roles in your metabolic narrative. How they interact is a fascinating tale that we'll delve into with the curiosity and rigor it deserves.

Nutrition, of course, can't be overlooked in discussions about metabolism. The macronutrients—carbohydrates, fats, and proteins—each influence your metabolism in unique ways, as do micronutrients, albeit on a subtler playing field. Hydration, too, is essential to your metabolic function, and understanding this relationship is critical.

Intermittent fasting has become a buzzword, and for good reason, but it's not a one-size-fits-all approach. We'll dissect the benefits, the different methods available, and also the cautions one should consider. The goal isn't just to inform but to give you the discernment needed to make choices aligned with your personal health panorama.

The gut, soon revealed to be the metropolis of metabolic activity, requires nurturing through a diet specifically tailored for its health. Probiotics and prebiotics are more than just trendy terms—they're tools at your disposal for metabolic harmony.

And for those of you thinking that deprivation or grueling exercise are the only solutions, rest easy. We'll explore the indispensability of sleep, the balancing act of exercising for metabolism without overdoing it, and how tracking progress and forming sustainable habits factor into real, long-term success.

What's importantly unique about this program is customization. This book isn't about following a rigid plan—it's about adapting principles to fit your life, your body, and your health conditions. Guidance from health professionals, understanding your body's cues and needs, and incorporating success strategies into your personal plan, all make up the fabric of this metabolic tapestry.

You'll read real-life stories to fuel your inspiration and tackle challenges like eating out and managing social events without derailing your progress. You'll also learn to recognize common pitfalls to avoid, how to cope with setbacks, and incredibly, how metabolic reset goes beyond weight loss, touching upon improved energy levels, mental clarity, and longevity.

By the end, you'll not just understand your metabolism; you'll have the skills and knowledge to respect it, nurture it, and reset it. This book is your map, your companion, and your resource, pointing toward a healthier, more energized you. So let's get started. Your metabolic reset journey begins now.

Chapter 1

Understanding Metabolism

As we pivot from the introduction and embark on this transformative journey, let's focus on one of the most bandied-about terms in the health and fitness realm: metabolism. It's a word that's often tossed around at the gym, in diet circles, and all over social media, but what does it actually encompass?

What Is Metabolism?

Metabolism, simply put, is the complex web of biological processes that convert food and beverages into energy. This ongoing chemical symphony allows your body to breathe, circulate blood, regulate temperature, and repair cells, amongst a myriad of other tasks. It's the engine of your body's car, and just like cars, some engines run more efficiently than others.

Now that we've opened the door to a healthier you, let's unravel one of the most thrown around yet misunderstood concepts in the health and wellness arena: metabolism. In simplest terms, metabolism is akin to an engine in your body, humming along throughout the day and night, converting food and stored energy into the fuel that powers everything from your thoughts to your marathon training.

At its core, metabolism encompasses all the chemical reactions in your body's cells that convert nutrients from the food you eat into vital energy. This energy isn't merely for movement; it's the currency your body uses for all its functions — repairing cells, breathing, circulating blood, and everything in between. It's the unseen laborer toiling tirelessly behind the scenes to ensure your body operates optimally.

Understanding your metabolism is more than just knowing about the food-to-energy process; it's about grasping how your body uses that energy. We can think of metabolism in two segments: catabolism, where larger molecules break down into energy, and anabolism, where that energy is used to construct components of cells like proteins and nucleic acids.

But it's not all about food. Metabolism has an intricate relationship with your body's fuel sources, hormones, and enzymes that help maintain balance — or homeostasis — in the body. Take the ebb and flow of your day; your metabolic rate isn't a constant speedometer reading. It shifts through the day, higher when you're active and dipping during sleep when the body goes into repair and recovery mode.

Many imagine metabolism as a switch that can be flicked on and off. In reality, it's more accurate to consider it a dial, with various factors turning the speed up or down. The idea of "boosting" metabolism is a bit of a misnomer. What we're really talking about is supporting and optimizing our body's intricate processes to operate smoothly, much like routine maintenance ensures a car engine runs effectively.

You might've heard phrases like 'metabolic rate' thrown around too. This term refers to how quickly your body burns calories at rest — known as the basal metabolic rate (BMR). And while two people might share the same height and weight, their BMR and the way their body processes energy could differ dramatically. It's a personalized number unique as a fingerprint.

When we speak of resetting the metabolism, we dive into the realm of influencing this basal metabolic rate and other metabolic processes in a way that supports weight loss and overall health. It's not about overhauling your body's innate systems but gently fine-tuning them to run more efficiently, particularly in the face of weight loss resistance or sluggish energy levels.

Resetting your metabolism isn't just about reducing calories or ramping up your exercise routine; it's a more nuanced approach that considers hormonal balances, nutritional intake, muscle mass, sleep patterns, and even stress levels. Each of these plays a vital role, acting as gears and cogs in your metabolic machine.

In this section, we'll keep it laser-focused on what metabolism is — steering clear of deeper discussions on related topics like myths or factors influencing metabolic rate — which we'll explore in detail in subsequent chapters. The clarity around the role of our metabolism lays the groundwork for the transformative strategies we'll cover for reshaping your health and eschewing unwanted pounds.

We now find ourselves at a critical junction in understanding metabolism's integral role in our body's ecosystem. With an appreciation for the complexity and beauty of our internal processes, we can move forward in pursuit of resetting and optimizing our metabolic engine. It's not about a quick fix, but aligning ourselves with our body's natural rhythm and fostering a healthy environment for it to thrive.

Factors That Influence Your Metabolic Rate

Now that we've explored what metabolism actually is, let's dive into the factors that can rev it up or slow it down - you're in for some eye-openers. Think of your metabolic rate like an engine; various elements can tune it up or throw a spanner in the works. Age, sex, and genetics surely play pivotal roles, setting the baseline of this metabolic machinery. They're the cards you're dealt, but that doesn't mean you can't shuffle the deck. Your daily habits and environs also have a say—yes, that's your lifestyle waving at you from the driver's seat. It's powerful stuff, knowing that you can turn the dial on your metabolism with a sprint or a standstill, with the foods you relish or the stress you manage. Don't get bogged down thinking about the uncontrollables in the genetic lottery. There's much at your behest, and we're here to harness that potential. Stick with me, and we'll tackle how to leverage your lifestyle to stoke the embers of your metabolic fire.

Age, Sex, and Genetics

Age, Sex, and Genetics are central to understanding the intricacies of metabolism, and how these factors play a significant role can't be understated. Age has a notorious reputation for slowing metabolic rate. It's not whimsy or fate; as we advance in years, our bodies tend to lose muscle mass and experience hormonal changes, both of which can decelerate the rate at which we burn calories. For those in the span of 20 to 70, this certainly indicates a continually shifting battle with the bulge. But fret not.

Understanding this can arm you with strategies to combat and reset your metabolism effectively.

When it comes to sex, men and women are not created equal – metabolically speaking. Generally, men possess more muscle mass and less body fat compared to women, which can translate into a higher resting metabolic rate. Ladies, this means the gents might have an easier time with weight management on paper, but there's more to the story than mere muscle bulk. Hormonal fluctuations throughout a woman's life, including the menstrual cycle and menopause, also interplay with metabolic speed, demanding a tailored approach for effective weight loss across genders.

Genetics can often seem like the wild card in the equation. Our genetic makeup has a profound influence on how our bodies process food and expend energy. Your genes can predispose you to certain traits, like a tendency to store fat in specific areas or a naturally lean physique. This doesn't imply that your genetic hand determines your metabolic fate. Instead, it highlights the importance of a personalized game plan for weight loss, one that considers your body's inherent tendencies.

It's vital to appreciate that these three factors — age, sex, and genetics — interconnect in complex ways to influence your metabolism. For instance, with age, men may experience a drop in testosterone levels, impacting muscle mass and metabolic rate. Meanwhile, women may see a shift in metabolic rate after childbirth or during menopause. It's a tangled web of internal systems interacting with each other, and a one-size-fits-all approach fails to address this complexity effectively.

But don't let this complexity dishearten you; it can actually empower you. Being mindful of the nuances shaped by age, sex, and genetics can guide you to more informed choices about diet, exercise, and lifestyle. It means recognizing that your metabolism is not static; it's as dynamic as life itself, changing and adapting as you age, and it can be influenced by your everyday choices.

For example, while you can't change your genetic code, you can certainly influence the expression of your genes through what's known as epigenetics. Lifestyle choices such as diet, exercise, and environmental exposures may alter the way your genes are expressed, potentially improving your metabolic health over time.

Women can harness the hormonal ebb and flow by tailoring their diet and exercise plans to different phases of their menstrual cycle or menopausal transition, optimizing metabolism even in the face of hormonal hurricanes. Similarly, men can offset testosterone decline with targeted resistance training that builds muscle mass and boosts metabolic rate. It's about playing to your personal physiological strengths while strategically mitigating the metabolic decline that comes with aging.

Let's not forget the serenity that comes from genetic acceptance. Sometimes, your genetics may predispose you to a particular metabolic pattern. This doesn't mean you're doomed to fight an uphill battle; rather, it means working smarter, not harder. Calibration to your body's characteristics is key, and success can be found when you align your metabolic reset efforts with your personal biological landscape.

Considering these factors — age, sex, and genetics — borders on imperative when devising a plan to reset your metabolism and shed unwanted weight. Ignoring them is akin to navigating without a map. With a nuanced understanding of these elements, you can craft a metabolic reset regimen that doesn't just aim for weight loss but also fits comfortably and sustainably within the tapestry of your life.

Enlightening yourself on these topics paves the way for a more successful and informed journey towards a metabolic reset. It's about personalized strategy rather than surrendering to a "one-size-fits-all" approach. Your metabolism isn't just your destiny; it's also a dynamic dance partner that you can learn to coordinate with harmoniously — even if the rhythm changes with age, the melody alters with sex, or the dance floor is set by your genetics.

Lifestyle and Environmental Factors

When it comes to resetting your metabolism and saying goodbye to those extra pounds, don't underestimate the power of lifestyle choices and the world around you. It's these very choices, from what you eat to how you sleep, and the environment you live in, that can make or break the efficacy of your metabolic reset. Let's dive into how these pieces of the puzzle fit together to shape your metabolic destiny.

First off, let's talk about diet. No, not those short-term crash diets that promise quick fixes, but nutritional choices that have a lasting impact. The stuff you choose to put on your plate each day isn't just fuel—it's information for your body. Eat a balanced diet rich in whole foods, fibers, and a variety of nutrients, and you'll be doing your metabolism a solid favor. Processed foods with lots of added sugars and fats? They can confuse your metabolic processes, bogging down the works.

Next comes the game-changer: physical activity. It goes beyond just burning calories. Regular physical activity subtly tweaks your metabolism toward efficiency, improving your body's ability to utilize energy. That doesn't mean you need to be a gym rat; even daily walks, taking the stairs, or a few yoga stretches can add up over time.

Don't overlook sleep either. It's not just about the quantity but also the quality. A restful night is like hitting the reset button on your body's stress levels. Poor sleep can cause havoc on your hormonal balance, influencing ghrelin and leptin, those pesky hormones that control appetite and can lead your metabolism astray.

Don't forget hydration! The simplicity of water is often understated. Drink enough of it, and your metabolism flows more smoothly. Dehydration can actually slow down many of the body's essential functions, including your metabolism. So, sip away—it's nature's drink of choice for metabolic health.

Meanwhile, environmental pollutants, chemicals, and even certain plastics can interfere with your body's natural hormonal functions. These endocrine disruptors found in everything from food packaging to cosmetics can be detrimental to your metabolic goals. Be mindful of your exposure and choose natural and eco-friendly products when possible.

Then there's the social and cultural environment. It's easy to underestimate the impact of our community and culture on eating habits. Being conscious of portion sizes, food choices, and the tendency to indulge in response to social cues is all part of crafting a responsive metabolic environment.

Finally, consider the significance of routine. A consistent sleep schedule, regular meal times, and a solid workout routine can entrench your metabolism in a rhythm that works for you rather than against you. Consistency can truly be one of your best allies in the fight to reset your metabolism.

Wrap all these factors up, and you have a powerful cocktail for influencing your metabolism. Each one may seem small on its own, but together they form a symphony of tweaks and adjustments that can amplify your metabolic function. It's a bit like having a well-oiled machine—keep it clean, maintained, and run it regularly, and it'll do wonders for you. It's time to give some serious thought to how you live, where you live, and the choices you make every day—they're not just about your waistline; they're about wellness writ large.

So, while genetics certainly play their part, remember that the baton is in your hands when it comes to lifestyle and environmental factors. Craft your lifestyle with intention, and your metabolism is more likely to follow suit, leading to that effective and sustainable weight loss you've been aiming for.

Myths About Metabolism

Now, let's dive into some common misconceptions that can really trip you up on your quest for a metabolic reset. Despite the wealth of information at our fingertips, the world of metabolism is shrouded in myths that steer many well-intentioned individuals off course. Uncovering the truth is pivotal. It'll not only save you from frustration but can also dramatically accelerate your progress toward weight loss.

One prevalent myth is that eating late at night is a surefire way to gain weight because your metabolism slows down while you sleep. However, the bigger picture revolves around total calorie intake over time, not the clock. It's not so much about when you eat, but *how much* you eat in relation to your daily energy expenditure. Fixating on meal timing can lead to unnecessary stress without impacting the scale.

Then there's the good old "fast metabolism" envy. Many believe some lucky folks are blessed with a metabolism so fast they can eat anything without gaining an ounce. While genetics play a role in metabolic rate, they aren't the sole determinant. Lifestyle choices and overall health have significant effects on your metabolism. So, bank on exercise and balanced nutrition rather than longing for genetic superpowers.

Another fable is the notion that skipping meals is a beneficial way to rev up your metabolism and spur weight loss. In truth, too often or extreme skipping can lead your body into a conservation mode where it becomes more efficient at using fewer calories. This doesn't mean you can't skip a meal if you're genuinely not hungry. Still, deliberate deprivation isn't the secret to metabolic success.

Ever heard someone say, "I can't lose weight because I have a slow metabolism"? It's a common refrain and a convenient escape. While metabolic rate varies between people, it's very rare for a "slow" metabolism to be the sole culprit for weight challenges. More often, a combination of diet, physical activity, and psychological factors play a much larger role.

How about "magic" metabolism-boosting foods? The concept that certain foods, like green tea or chili peppers, can significantly rev your metabolic engine has been overhyped. These foods might offer a tiny boost, but they're no substitute for the broader lifestyle changes needed to reset your metabolism effectively.

And don't even get me started on those who say metabolism is all downhill after 30. Yes, age can affect metabolic rate, but it's not the dramatic plunge some make it out to be. Keeping active and gaining muscle mass through strength training can offset many of the reductions in metabolism attributed to aging.

Remember the adage that muscle burns more calories than fat, so loading up on muscle will turn your body into a calorie-torching furnace? There's truth to muscle being more metabolically active than fat, but the difference isn't as vast as gym lore suggests. Building muscle is excellent for overall health and metabolism, but expecting it to miraculously evaporate excess calories is wishful thinking.

Lastly, many believe that weight gain is an inevitable result of a sluggish metabolism. Yet, metabolism is only part of the weight gain story. Excess caloric intake and a sedentary lifestyle are typically the primary contributors. Blaming metabolism alone neglects the power of proactive change in diet and physical activity.

Debunking these myths equips you with a clearer path to reengineering your metabolic health. By focusing on factual information, you can craft a more effective plan that will yield the results you're hoping for. Stay informed, stay persistent, and watch as that recalibrated metabolism works with you, not against you, on this journey to better health.

Chapter 2

The Signs of a Slow Metabolism

As we peel back the layers of metabolism's complexity, it's crucial to spot the tell-tale signs that yours might be lagging. Are you often tired, even though you've got a full night's sleep? Perhaps you've noticed that your jeans are feeling a bit too cozy, or your weight's creeping up, despite your eating habits remaining unchanged. Skin feeling dry, brittle nails, or hair loss can be subtle whispers of an underlying metabolic sluggishness. And let's not forget the mental fog that sweeps in uninvited, staying for longer than we'd want – these are all nudges from your body, hinting that it's time to tune into your metabolic health. Sure, a slow metabolism isn't the villain in every weight loss story, but understanding its signals is a powerful step toward turning the tides in your favor. So, let's dive in and decode the messages your body is sending, ensuring that no symptom is lost in translation, and set the stage for the revitalizing metabolic reset that awaits.

Recognizing the Symptoms

As we've seen, metabolism is the powerhouse of the body, driving dozens of bodily processes every single second. Now, if you suspect your own metabolic engine might not be firing on all cylinders, paying attention to certain signs is critical. Recognizing the symptoms of a slow metabolism can serve as the catalyst for change and the first step towards a healthier, more vibrant life.

First off, let's talk about weight gain. If the number on the scale has started to creep up despite your eating habits remaining the same, a slowed metabolism could be the sneak thief. It's like your body, once a symphony of energy-burning efficiency, has suddenly toned down the tempo, and now those calories aren't turning into energy quite as fast as they used to.

But hey, it's not all about weight. Feeling tired more often than a sloth on a lazy Sunday? That could be your slow metabolism not producing enough oomph to keep you energized through the day. It's like your body is conserving every scrap of energy, doling it out sparingly rather than with the generosity it once had.

Are you always reaching for a sweater even when others are comfortable? This could signal a downshift in your metabolism. Your internal thermostat isn't generating enough heat, leaving you feeling cold when no one else seems to be reaching for extra layers.

Then there's the conundrum of not-so-regular bowel movements. A sluggish metabolism can lead to a sluggish digestive system, making constipation an unwelcome but very telling guest. It's as if your body's conveyor belt of digestion is moving at snail's pace, affecting everything from appetite to stomach comfort.

And when it comes to your favorite jeans not fitting the way they used to, well, it's not just about the weight. A slower metabolism can lead to increased fat storage, particularly around the midsection. Your body, rather than using fat as fuel, is more likely to store it like a squirrel hoarding nuts for winter.

Mood swings and brain fog? Yep, a slow metabolism might be meddling with your cognitive function and emotional well-being. When your metabolic rate takes a nosedive, it can affect everything from your ability to concentrate to your overall mood. It's as if your brain is trying to jog through molasses, making every thought and every decision feel that much more laborious.

Let's not forget the state of your hair and nails. Brittle nails and hair loss can signal a lack of essential nutrients making their way to these areas due to a plodding metabolism. Your once luscious locks and strong nails need a steady supply of nutrients, and a slow metabolism can interrupt that nourishing flow.

Sleep patterns can also become erratic. If you find yourself struggling to catch a good night's rest, it might be connected to metabolic imbalances, particularly in blood sugar levels, which can lead to both insomnia and that groggy feeling after a night of unrestful sleep. It's like your internal clock has lost its rhythm, leaving you tossing and turning instead of peacefully slumbering.

Lastly, if healing from injuries or recovering from exercise is taking longer than it used to, this too can be a sign of metabolic sluggishness. A robust metabolism helps repair and rebuild, but when it's slow, all of these processes, including recovery, get delayed. Imagine your body's repair crew moving at the speed of a tortoise—this is what happens when your metabolism isn't in top form.

Understanding these signs is paramount. They're not just complaints or random occurrences; they could be your body signaling for help, letting you know it's time to reevaluate how you fuel and maintain your metabolic machinery. Identifying a slow metabolism is the first step, but fear not—once you're aware, you can take the reins and steer yourself towards metabolic mastery.

How Slow Metabolism Affects Your Body and Mind

Understanding the splash a slow metabolism can make in your life is kind of like realizing that your once zippy smartphone has started to lag. Sure, you might not give it much thought until you need it to perform swiftly. And it's that sluggishness, not just an annoyance but a sign that something's not quite right beneath the surface. Slow metabolism doesn't just settle for dimming your energy levels; it reaches out, threading its way into various aspects of your health and mental well-being.

Let's paint a picture here: imagine the frustration when you're doing everything 'by the book', but the scale seems stuck. That's a hallmark struggle for those battling a creeping metabolism. Excess weight, particularly around the midsection, can be stubborn. And it's not just about aesthetics, either. It's a visible sign that your body's fuel-burning engine is idling when it should be revving.

But the reach of a slow metabolism extends beyond your waistline. Ever felt like you're wading through molasses all day? That fatigue that clings despite a full night's sleep might be your body hinting at a metabolic slowdown. It's not just a lack of energy—it's a lack of energy production. And with less energy, simple tasks become herculean efforts. It's the physiological equivalent of trying to climb a staircase with weight tied to your ankles.

Then there's the cold. Not just a winter chill, but a near constant companion. If you're always layering up while others are comfortable, your internal thermostat might be showing the effects of a sluggish metabolism, struggling to generate enough heat to keep you toasty.

Your mental fog might also be thicker than a morning mist. A slow metabolism can take the sharpness out of your cognition, clouding your concentration and memory. It's as if your brain's circuits are flickering, creating an environment where focus is a fleeting commodity, and cognitive function seems to be running a step behind.

On a cellular level, slow metabolism can be like a dimmer switch on your body's repair processes. Cellular regeneration and healing might take an unwanted hiatus, leaving you wondering why the cut on your finger is taking a 'lazy Sunday' approach to healing.

And how's your mood sitting with you? If you find that you're more downcast than usual, it might not just be circumstance. The delicate dance of hormones and neurotransmitters in your body can be influenced by metabolic shifts, potentially turning you into a bit more of a melancholy soul than you're used to being.

But it's not just about feeling blue. A slow metabolism can nudge hormones related to stress and anxiety into the spotlight. It's like your body constantly thinks it's in the middle of a bad traffic jam, pumping out stress signals when you just need to relax.

Your hair and skin can also whisper secrets about your metabolic pace. Dry, brittle hair and lackluster skin may not just be about needing a new shampoo or moisturizer; they could be the banners revealing the impact of a metabolism that's lost its spark.

Finally, delve deeper and you'll find your body's harmony at risk. Digestion can turn into a tumultuous affair, with a slow metabolism leading to bloating and constipation. It's your body saying, "Hey, I'm not processing this stuff as quickly as I should be."

Why does all this matter? Because it's not just about weight. It's about the symphony of your overall health playing in beautiful unison. Understanding the far-reaching effects of a slow metabolism can empower you to fine-tune your body's orchestra, transforming each silent whisper of dysfunction into a powerful ally for vitality. And that's precisely what's on the menu when we talk about resetting your metabolism—it's a lot more than shedding pounds; it's about rediscovering the rhythm that keeps you thriving.

When to Seek Medical Advice

As you've learned to spot the signals of a sluggish metabolism, it's crucial to know when to transition from self-help tactics to seeking professional guidance. If you find the weighing scale stubbornly unmoving, or if growing fatigue is your constant shadow despite adequate rest, it might be time to raise the flag. Let's dive deeper into circumstances that merit the expertise of medical professionals.

First and foremost, if you're experiencing unexplained and persistent changes in weight that fly in defiance of your healthy habits and exercise routines, it could hint at underlying health issues. Your metabolism doesn't operate in isolation; it is interlinked with complex hormonal pathways that can sometimes go awry, and a healthcare provider can help navigate these complexities.

Secondly, stubborn fatigue isn't just a sign of too many late nights but could also be an indicator of metabolic distress. When your energy balance equation doesn't add up despite a well-managed diet and sleep cycle, there's potentially more to the story. A professional can conduct appropriate tests to pinpoint disorders such as hypothyroidism, which slow down your metabolism and sap your vigor.

Another red flag is intolerance to cold. If you find yourself layering up while others are comfortable, it could be more than just personal preference; it's possibly your metabolism signaling that it's unable to generate sufficient heat, a job intricately linked to thyroid function.

Mood fluctuations and brain fog also deserve your attention. While it's normal to experience the occasional blue day or a moment of forgetfulness, consistent spells could point towards metabolic imbalance influencing your neurological and psychological well-being. Seeking medical advice ensures you receive comprehensive care that looks beyond the scale and into your mental health.

Frequent muscle weakness or cramps can also be associated with metabolic issues. This is particularly worth noting if you're getting the right nutrients and staying hydrated. Muscles are metabolic powerhouses, and when they frequently protest, it's time to listen and consult with a healthcare provider to root out deficiencies or hormonal imbalances affecting muscle function.

If you notice changes in your hair or skin – perhaps your hair has become thinner, or your skin drier than the Sahara – your body might be signaling nutritional deficiencies or hormonal imbalances that require a closer look.

Metabolism is deeply connected to the delivery of nutrients to your body's tissues, and deviations in your external appearance can reflect internal turbulence.

Lastly, if you've fruitlessly tried various diet and exercise regimens with little to no success, it's safe to say an expert opinion might be the missing puzzle piece. Metabolic health is not a DIY project when roadblocks persist; professional advice can tailor a plan specific to your biology and needs.

Remember, consulting with a healthcare provider isn't a defeat; it's a smart strategic move. It's easy to get swayed by the overload of wellness advice that permeates our lives, but the assistance of a professional provides science-backed, individualized guidance. By partnering with a trusted medical expert, you take a crucial step towards resetting your metabolism and ushering in sustainable weight loss and overall health.

Considering the spectrum of symptoms that could signal the need for medical intervention, it's prudent to err on the side of caution. Timely professional advice can make the difference between spinning your wheels and advancing toward your health goals. Your journey towards a metabolic reset is uniquely yours, but it's wise to have a medical ally in your corner to navigate any hiccups along the way.

So, as you charter the waters of resetting your metabolism, keep an eye out for these signals and be proactive in seeking medical counsel. They are the lighthouses guiding you to safer shores, ensuring that you reach your destination of metabolic health armed with the right support, rather than journeying in treacherous waters alone.

Chapter 3

The Science of Metabolic Reset

As we've explored the intricacies of metabolism and the signals of a slow one, it's time we dive into the transformative world of metabolic reset. This isn't just a fleeting trend; it's rooted deeply in science and steeped in our bodies' incredible capacity for adaptation. That's right, our bodies are dynamic systems, not fixed machines, and understanding this is pivotal to reinvigorating our metabolic health.

Some think of metabolism as a predetermined engine speed, but think again. Metabolic adaptation is your body's natural ability to adjust its metabolic rate in response to various conditions. When we talk about "resetting" metabolism, we're essentially referring to reprogramming this internal process to function more efficiently and effectively.

It's essential to get to the heart of the matter: hormones. These biochemical messengers are the maestros orchestrating the ebb and flow of your metabolic processes. Two players deserve mention here: insulin and glucagon, which act like a dance duo managing blood sugar levels, while thyroid hormones play a powerful role in regulating metabolic rate. It's a delicate balance, and when it's off, it's like a well-choreographed dance turning into a freestyle of awkward moves.

But it's not just about individual hormones; it's about the complex inter-play between them and other physiological systems. A metabolic reset aims to fine-tune this hormonal conversation, sharpening the body's ability to respond to metabolic demands. It's akin to upgrading the dialogue within a sophisticated network, ensuring messages are clear and responses are prompt.

Now here's a thought: the process of metabolic reset isn't a one-time event. Instead, it's a series of strategic, sustainable changes that encourage your body to adapt over time. This is where the excitement lies—you're not just a passive bystander in your health journey; you're the director, and you can indeed coax your metabolism back to a more sprightly state.

Perhaps you're puzzled about how all of this works? Well, we'll delve into nutrition, fasting, exercise, and more in-depth later. But understand this — a metabolic reset isn't about depleting your body; it's about replenishing and reinvigorating it. It's about taking control and directing your body toward a state where weight loss isn't a struggle but a natural consequence of a finely tuned metabolic engine.

Consider the possibility that, despite your current metabolic state, you can ignite change. You've ridden the waves of trendy diets and fast-fix solutions, only to circle back to frustration. Those days can be a thing of the past. Picture yourself stepping into a future where you manage your metabolism rather than it managing you. The power lies within the grasp of your hand—it is yours for the taking!

Keep in mind, though, that the pursuit of metabolic reset isn't a mere adjustment of the thermostat — it's a remodeling of the entire heating system. And like any significant renovation, you'll need the right tools and blueprints, which we'll provide as you move through this metabolic masterclass. By now, you understand that metabolic rate is not a victim to fate; your daily choices and practices have immense power to reshape it.

So let's gear up—not with apprehension but with anticipation—for the revelations and methods that won't just reset your metabolism but redefine your relationship with your body. It's about unlocking the potential that has been dormant for far too long. Get ready to step into a journey that's not just about losing weight but about gaining a renewed sense of vitality and well-being that can last a lifetime.

With a solid grasp of the science behind metabolic reset, you're poised at the threshold of transformation. Hold tight to the principles we've covered, because as we move forward, every step, every chapter builds upon this foundational knowledge, bringing you closer to the metabolic health you're striving for. It's time to redefine what's possible, one metabolic reset at a time.

Introduction to Metabolic Adaptation

Having brushed up on the basics of metabolism and identifying the tell-tale signs of a slowdown, it's time to dive deeper. We're embarking on a journey through the intricate dance of metabolic adaptation – a concept pivotal to understanding the science of resetting your metabolism. Think of your metabolism not as a static entity, but as a dynamic and responsive orchestra, fine-tuning its performance according to the demands of its environment.

At its core, metabolic adaptation refers to the body's ability to alter its metabolic rate – the tempo at which it expends energy – to best suit its current state. It's the body's innate tactic for survival, honed over millennia, allowing us to navigate a landscape that was once scarce with food. Perhaps frustratingly for many, this primal survival mechanism can also mean that our bodies become all too efficient, storing energy as fat when we'd prefer it to rev up the metabolic engines and burn it off.

In essence, adaptability is a hallmark of life itself, and your metabolism is no exception. When you cut calories or ramp up exercise, your body isn't just passively watching the show – it's an active participant, adjusting your energy expenditure to accommodate these changes. Imagine you're driving a car: As the road conditions change, you shift gears to maintain speed and efficiency. Your metabolism does much the same, albeit to preserve balance within your body. It responds to how much you eat, what you eat, and how you burn energy through a complex interplay of hormones and cellular signals – but more on that in the following sections.

We often see metabolic adaptation in the form of a weight loss plateau – your body's tendency to 'hold onto' weight after initial success. This isn't a sign that you've done anything wrong; rather, it's your body's natural braking system kicking in. It's adapting to your new lifestyle, trying to conserve what it considers precious fuel. The trick, however, lies in outsmarting this ancient mechanism to achieve and sustain weight loss, which is precisely the goal we aim for with a metabolic reset.

Understanding this concept is key to resetting your metabolism. It helps in realizing why crash diets or sudden bursts of high-intensity workouts can't offer sustainable results. Metabolic adaptation doesn't happen overnight, and neither does resetting it. It requires a methodical approach that nudges the metabolism gently and persuasively, encouraging it to adjust its set-point – the weight your body naturally gravitates towards – to a healthier level.

What's equally interesting is the role individual differences play in metabolic adaptation. Factors such as genetics, age, and body composition mean that everyone's metabolism will respond differently to changes. This is why personalization is essential; there's no one-size-fits-all answer to metabolic health.

The coming chapters will outline how various components, such as hormones, nutrition, fasting, sleep, and exercise influence metabolic adaptation. They will provide strategic insights needed to effectively reset your metabolism. We'll explore how to coax the metabolism into increasing its resting rate, essentially turning up the dial on your daily calorie burn without the need for dramatic lifestyle upheavals. It's about making smarter, scientifically-backed choices that work with your body, not against it.

So, as we delve into the fascinating science of metabolic adaptation, keep an open mind. Perhaps past attempts at weight loss haven't considered the adaptable nature of your metabolism – but with this new understanding, you're better equipped to embark on a transformation that's not just effective but sustainable too. By learning to facilitate rather than fight against metabolic adaptation, you're setting the stage for a truly transformative metabolic reset.

Remember, as you read on, that the ultimate goal is not just shedding pounds; it's fostering a lifelong synergy with your body's rhythms. A reset metabolism isn't merely about a lower number on the scales – it's the foundation of vibrant energy levels, a thriving body, and a more empowered you. Now, let's begin the rewarding process of tapping into your body's amazing ability to adapt and recalibrate for improved metabolic health.

The Role of Hormones in Metabolic Health

Let's talk about the maestros of our body's metabolic orchestra—the hormones. These chemical messengers are crucial in instructing our bodies how to function, especially when it comes to metabolic health. To reset your metabolism effectively, you need to understand these players and how they can be tuned to perform at their best.

Hormones are kind of like the software that directs our bodily functions. They travel through the bloodstream, delivering messages to different parts of the body to regulate metabolism and other physiological processes. One misstep in this communication, and you've got metabolic discord. Imagine trying to listen to a concerto where the instruments are out of sync—it's not pretty. And it's not just about one or two hormones; it's about the balance and harmony of the entire system.

Let's take insulin, for instance. This hormone is like the body's accountant, carefully managing how much sugar stays in the blood and how much gets stored for later. Too much of it hanging around, and you might be dealing with insulin resistance—a primary villain in the metabolic mayhem that can lead to weight gain and type 2 diabetes.

Ghrelin and leptin are another hormone duo that deserves a spotlight. These are the Hunger Games' main commentators, with ghrelin ringing the dinner bell and leptin telling you it's time to push the plate away. If their signaling is off, you might find yourself snacking non-stop, like during a movie marathon with unlimited popcorn. It's easy to see why keeping them in check is essential for managing appetite and, by extension, weight.

You've also got your thyroid hormones. These are your body's thermostat, controlling how fast or slow your metabolic engine runs. A sluggish thyroid can leave you feeling tired and cold, while an overactive one can turn the heat up too much. And just like a sensitive thermostat, the ideal settings for your thyroid can be unique to you.

Corticosteroids, particularly cortisol, are hormones that dictate your body's response to stress, among other things. Sure, a little stress can be a kickstarter in the morning, but chronic stress can lead cortisol to whisper sweet nothings to your fat cells, encouraging them to hang around, particularly around your midsection.

Sex hormones like estrogen and testosterone aren't just about reproductive health—they're part of the metabolic conversation, too. When these are out of balance, it's not uncommon to see fluctuations in energy levels, muscle mass, and fat distribution.

So, you might be wondering, what can we do about all this hormonal interplay? For starters, you can eat right, get enough sleep, manage stress better, and move your body. Simple changes can speak volumes to your hormones, coaxing them into a harmonious balance that supports a healthy metabolism. There's no need for drastic measures; even subtle lifestyle tweaks can lead to significant metabolic improvements.

Remember, your body's ability to effectively manage weight is highly influenced by the intricate dance of hormones. If any of these key players miss a step, it can throw your whole metabolic rhythm off balance. We'll delve into specifics in later chapters, especially when discussing how insulin and thyroid hormones directly affect your metabolic rate. However, keep this holistic view in mind: weight loss isn't just about calories and exercise. It's also about optimizing the endocrine system, the very system that guides a vast array of metabolic processes.

With this knowledge, you're better equipped to understand the advice we're about to dive into in the following chapters. When we eventually discuss insulin and thyroid hormones, you'll know these aren't isolated factors but part of a bigger, complex system that can be gently steered in the right direction to help you achieve metabolic nirvana. Think of it as conducting your body's metabolic symphony to create a balance that resonates with health and vitality—a concept that's music to our ears.

Insulin and Glucagon

These two hormones are like the yin and yang of blood sugar management and metabolic regulation. They're secret agents that your pancreas dispatches to maintain the delicate balance of glucose in your bloodstream, which is crucial, especially when you're reprogramming your metabolism to shed some pounds.

Insulin, think of it as the storage guru, springs into action when your blood sugar levels spike post-meal. It tells your cells, "Hey, we've got energy here! Let's take this glucose and store it or use it, stat!" Cells fling open their doors, letting sugar in to be either used as fuel or stored as glycogen in the liver and muscles. If there's still sugar to spare, insulin goes ahead and converts it into fat. That's its way of keeping blood sugar levels from turning into a rollercoaster.

On the flip side, when your sugar reserves dip too low, glucagon picks up the torch. It nudges your liver to convert stored glycogen back into glucose and release it into your bloodstream. This back-and-forth dance between insulin and glucagon ensures your cells have a steady stream of fuel—not too much, not too little.

Let's talk about why these hormones are VIPs in the weight loss party. If your insulin levels are always high because you're snacking on carbs around the clock, for instance, your body's fat-burning processes slow down. It's like constantly filling your gas tank; if you don't drive enough, you won't need to burn off that fuel. Over time, your cells might also start ignoring insulin's calls—this is insulin resistance, and it's a straight-up metabolism mess-up.

Now, if you're thinking, "So, I just need to lower my insulin to lose weight, right?" Hang on a minute—it's more nuanced than that. While keeping your insulin levels low helps, you must also ensure that glucagon is doing its thing correctly. Knowing when and how to influence these hormones can make or break your metabolic reset journey.

How does one find that hormonal harmony? Well, it starts with the right diet and timing. When you eat foods that cause less of an insulin spike—like fiber-rich veggies, healthy fats, and lean proteins—you're giving insulin a bit of a break. And when you space out your meals or try intermittent fasting, you give glucagon a chance to swing into action.

You might be thinking, "But I love my pasta and bread!" Fear not! It's about balance and understanding that not all carbs are created equal. Whole grains can be part of a healthy diet, but in the right portions and at the right times. Meals shouldn't turn into an all-you-can-eat sugar buffet for your blood.

Exercise is another key player. Moving your body increases insulin sensitivity, which means your cells respond better to insulin, and you don't need as much of it to lower blood sugar levels. Plus, working out helps burn through glycogen stores, making room for glucagon to fill them back up. It's a fantastic cycle that keeps the metabolism revved up.

Finally, there's the sleep factor. Poor sleep can lead to hormonal mayhem, making your insulin sluggish and less effective. Yes, the secret sauce includes hitting the sack for a solid 7-9 hours each night to keep insulin and glucagon performing their best.

Understanding how insulin and glucagon work can seem daunting, but it's essential for harnessing their power for weight loss and overall metabolic health. In upcoming chapters, we'll dive deeper into foods, fasting, and lifestyle tweaks that help these hormones help you. But for now, remember: mastering metabolism requires a duet, not a solo performance, and insulin and glucagon are the lead singers in this band. Keep their harmony, and you're on your way to a finely tuned metabolic masterpiece.

Thyroid Hormones

Let's zero in on one of the most critical players in your metabolic symphony: thyroid hormones. These little molecules are like the conductors, ensuring that the metabolic processes within your cells stay in perfect tempo. Their essential role might not be new information, but understanding their power can provide striking insights into resetting and improving your metabolism.

Thyroid hormones come in two main forms – thyroxine (T4) and tri-iodothyronine (T3). Your thyroid gland, sitting unassumingly at the front of your neck, pumps out these hormones, which then embark on a journey through your bloodstream to virtually every cell in your body. Their mission is critical: to regulate the speed at which your cells work, in other words, your metabolic rate.

It's a fascinating process, really. T4 is like a storage hormone; it's not particularly active in this form, but it acts as a reserve ready to be transformed into the more potent T3 when the body needs it. Enzymes in your organs, like the liver and kidneys, then take T4 and convert it into T3, which proceeds to stoke the metabolic fires.

Why is a well-regulated thyroid so crucial for weight management? It's because your thyroid hormones influence various metabolic functions. They control how your body burns calories, how you process carbohydrates and fats, and even the rate at which your heart beats. When the thyroid is out of tune, it can throw your metabolic harmony into disarray, potentially slowing down your weight loss efforts despite your best diet and exercise plans.

And here's the kicker – an underactive thyroid, or hypothyroidism, isn't uncommon. This condition stealthily slows metabolism, leading to fatigue, weight gain, and a host of other symptoms that can be easily overlooked or attributed to other causes. Getting your thyroid hormone levels checked is a simple yet pivotal step in identifying whether this is a hurdle in your metabolic reset journey.

But it's not only about the quantity of these hormones; their function can also be hampered by various factors. Stress, nutritional deficiencies (particularly iodine and selenium), and exposure to environmental toxins can all affect how effective thyroid hormones are in doing their job. This means that beyond the hormonal quantity, we must also focus on supporting the factors that influence the hormone's efficiency.

As integral as thyroid hormones are, popping synthetic hormones isn't always the answer. The key lies in supporting your body's natural ability to produce these hormones and convert T4 to T3 efficiently. Nutrition plays a starring role in this. Foods rich in iodine, such as seafood and seaweed, and selenium, found in Brazil nuts and sunflower seeds, can support thyroid health. Regular intake of these micronutrients can help fine-tune your hormonal orchestra.

Exercise, too, deserves a highlight. By engaging in regular physical activity, you encourage your body to be more sensitive to thyroid hormones. It's like upgrading the communication system within your body, ensuring that when thyroid hormones send out the signal to ramp up metabolism, your cells are quick to respond.

Now, let's not forget that excess thyroid hormones can be as problematic as a deficiency, leading to hyperthyroidism, where your metabolism could be running too hot. This might sound like a weight loss dream, but it's a health nightmare, potentially leading to severe consequences such as muscle breakdown and heart problems. Balance, as always, is the name of the game.

Remember, the goal here isn't to artificially crank up your hormones but to restore your body's natural rhythm, allowing for sustainable weight management. It's about rejuvenating your cellular metabolism to work in favor of your health and vitality. Managing thyroid health is one of the finest tunes you can compose on the path to metabolic harmony and a life lived to its fullest potential.

Chapter 4

The Role of Nutrition in Metabolism

Now that we've demystified metabolism and unearthed the influences of hormones, let's chew over the profound impact nutrition has on your body's metabolic orchestra. Sure, you've heard the old adage that 'you are what you eat,' but let's dig a bit deeper—because it's not just about the calories you consume, it's about the quality. The right balance of macronutrients—those carbs, fats, and proteins—can gear up your metabolism like a well-oiled machine, while the neglected micronutrients are the unsung heroes, fine-tuning your bodily functions. And water? It's not just about quenching thirst; hydration is pivotal for metabolic efficiency. It's time to give your body the fuel it needs to rev up the engine and keep it purring like a luxury sports car, rather than sputtering along in a clunker. Embrace the power of good nutrition, and watch as it transforms your metabolic health, ushering in a new era of energy and weight loss.

Macronutrients and Metabolism

As you've settled into the flow of unlocking the mysteries of metabolism, let's zoom in on the muscular trio: carbohydrates, fats, and proteins—our trusty macronutrients. Picture them as the crucial keys that start the engine of your body's metabolic car. Carbs are like the quick-burning fuel, great for getting you off the starting line fast. But don't let fats fool you; they're like high-density fuel pellets, storing massive energy reserves for the long haul, ensuring you don't just stop in your tracks. Proteins? Well, they're the body's pit crew, constantly in repair and rebuild mode, maintaining your metabolic machinery. It's not just about slashing calories; it's about leveraging the precise balance of these macronutrients to stoke your metabolic fire. What you're really aiming for is to teach your metabolism to be nimble, to switch gears between fuel sources with the elegance of a top-tier athlete. Transform your fuel intake, and you transform your body's ability to burn that fuel. This isn't just about shedding pounds; it's about shaping a metabolism that works for you, not against you. Remember, shifting into a high-gear metabolism doesn't mean revving up to redline; it means fine-tuning your nutritional intake for peak performance and endurance on this weight-loss race.

Carbohydrates and their role in metabolism is a tale as old as time. Often misunderstood, vilified, or adored, these macronutrients are fundamental to energy production and overall health. What really matters is the type of carbs you're indulging in and how they fit into your metabolic reset.

First, let's demystify what carbohydrates are. Simply put, they're organic compounds comprised of sugars, starches, and fiber, which the body breaks down into glucose—the primary source of energy for your cells. But here's where it gets interesting: not all carbs are created equal. You've probably heard the terms' simple' and 'complex,' and they're pivotal when resetting your metabolism.

Simple carbs, found in foods like candy or pastries, are quick energy sources. They spike your blood sugar, leading to an inevitable crash. Now, contrast that with complex carbs—found in vegetables, whole grains, and legumes—which are metabolically friendly. They break down slowly, releasing energy over time, keeping hunger pangs at bay and preventing blood sugar spikes.

When considering a metabolic reset, you might wonder how carbohydrates fit into the picture. To put it bluntly, they're essential. But the trick lies in selecting high-fiber, nutrient-dense carbohydrates that don't just fuel your body but also support digestive health, essential for a thriving metabolism.

But let's not ignore the elephant in the room—low-carb diets. They can be useful, especially in the short term for rapid weight loss. Reducing carb intake can lead to lower insulin levels and increased fat burning. However, the goal here is a metabolic reset, not a quick fix. Profound and sustainable health transformation requires a balanced approach to carb consumption—not their complete elimination.

Don't underestimate the importance of fiber, a type of carbohydrate, in metabolic regulation. Fiber doesn't just travel through your system, ushering out waste; it also regulates the usage of sugars, helping to keep hunger and blood sugar in check. Think of fiber as your metabolism's calm, reliable best friend, always there to smooth out the rough edges.

Now, indulge me as we talk timing. The timing of your carb intake can subtly influence your metabolism. Consuming the majority of your day's carbs around your workouts — when your body is primed to utilize them for recovery and energy replenishment — may prove beneficial. It's like syncing your carbs to your body's own rhythm.

It's not just about what and when; it's also about how much. Portion control is a guiding principle in a balanced metabolic reset. And yes, that includes carbs. If you load your plate with a mountain of pasta every night, you'll sabotage your efforts. Still, a controlled amount can provide the necessary energy without halting progress.

Let's not forget that a carb-restricted diet is a strain on discipline and often isn't realistic in the long term. Balancing carb intake allows for more sustainable habits, meaning you're more likely to stay on track with your metabolic reset. You'll be rewiring your body to use energy efficiently, rather than just cutting out an energy source altogether.

In short, the key to weaving carbohydrates into the fabric of your metabolic reset lies in choosing high-quality, high-fiber carbs, consuming them in moderation, and aligning their intake with your body's natural energy needs. Carbs aren't the enemy. Mismanagement of carbs is. Let's use them intelligently to refuel the body, reinvigorate the metabolism, and rebuild our relationship with food for lasting weight loss and health benefits.

Fats have too often been demonized in the world of nutrition. Yet, they're a vital macronutrient, playing a central role in your metabolic health. Let's dispel the myths and get to the heart of how the right kinds of fats can transform your metabolism.

First things first, fats are not the enemy. They're essential for the absorption of fat-soluble vitamins like A, D, E, and K, and they provide the body with a concentrated source of energy. Fats are involved in a multitude of body functions, from cell membrane integrity to hormone production. When you reset your metabolism, you're not cutting out fats; you're choosing them wisely.

There's a buzz around certain types of fats, particularly Omega-3 and Omega-6 fatty acids, and for good reason. Omega-3 fats, found in fish, flaxseed, and walnuts, for instance, are known for their anti-inflammatory properties and vital role in brain health. Omega-6 fats are also essential but need to be consumed in balance with Omega-3s to maintain optimal health.

But wait, what about saturated fats? We've been told to avoid them at all costs, but the truth is more nuanced. Your body needs some saturated fats from animal and plant sources, but the key is moderation. Overconsumption can lead to health problems, but in the right amounts, they're an important part of a nutrient-dense diet that fuels metabolic health.

Then there are trans fats, the real villains in the world of fats. These manufactured fats, found in processed and fried foods, are associated with an increased risk of chronic diseases and should be avoided to maintain a healthy metabolism.

Perhaps you've heard of the ketogenic diet, a high-fat, low-carb regimen that has many evangelists. This diet flips the traditional food pyramid on its head, claiming to reset your metabolism by forcing the body into a state of ketosis. While it's had remarkable results for some, it's not a one-size-fits-all solution. The takeaway? Your body can adapt to using fats as a primary fuel source.

If you're eyeing those avocados and nuts, you're on the right track. These foods offer healthy monounsaturated fats, which can help to lower bad cholesterol and reduce heart disease risk. They're also incredibly satisfying, helping to control appetite and prevent overeating—a boon for weight management.

You might have queries about how much fat you should be consuming. It's not about eating spoonfuls of coconut oil or gorging on bacon—your fat intake should be in alignment with your overall calorie needs and health goals. Generally, fats should make up about 20-35% of your daily calorie intake, but these needs can vary.

And don't forget about cooking! The way you prepare your foods can vastly affect the health benefits of fats. Opting for cooking methods like baking, steaming, or grilling, rather than frying, can help maintain the integrity of the fats you eat. Additionally, choosing high-quality, minimally processed oils, like extra virgin olive oil, can add to your metabolic success.

Ultimately, fats have a profound impact on your metabolic reset journey. Incorporating a diverse array of healthy fats can aid in resetting your metabolism, supporting weight loss, and enhancing overall well-being. It's about quality, balance, and making informed choices that support the complex, beautiful machine that is your body. As you continue to explore the role of nutrition in metabolism, remember that fats are a friend, not a foe, when chosen wisely and consumed in moderation.

Proteins – they're more than just fuel for muscles or the stuff bodybuilders obsess over. When we think about resetting metabolism for weight loss, overlooking the power of protein is like trying to cycle with a flat tire – you're not getting anywhere fast. Dive into why proteins are crucial and how they rev up your metabolic engine, ensuring that each bite you take translates into a healthier, leaner you.

Now, proteins are the body's building blocks – we're talking about muscle, bone, enzymes, and hormones. Sure, you know protein is important, but are you aware of how it directly affects your metabolism? It's not just about quantity; the type of protein matters too. Your body uses more energy to digest proteins compared to carbs or fats. This process, known as the thermic effect of food, means that protein can give your metabolism a nudge just by you enjoying your meal.

But wait, before you go grilling a steak the size of a hubcap, let's talk balance and moderation. High-quality proteins – think lean meats, fish, eggs, dairy, and plant-based sources like beans and lentils – should be enjoyed in the right amounts. And unlike fats and carbs, your body doesn't stash away protein for a rainy day. That means, to keep that metabolic engine purring, you need to replenish your protein stores regularly, without overdoing it.

Ever heard of amino acids? They're the VIPs in the world of protein, especially when it comes to weight loss. Essential amino acids – the ones your body can't make on its own – are key to maintaining muscle mass, which burns more calories at rest than fat does. When your diet is rich in these essential amino acids, you're supporting your metabolism's fat-burning capabilities, even as you cut calories.

Planning your protein intake throughout the day also plays into the metabolic reset equation. No, you don't need a degree in nutrition to figure this out. It's about ensuring each meal and snack has a protein element to maintain muscle mass and keep hunger at bay, which can prevent overeating. That's a win-win for your waistline and your metabolic rate.

Another metabolic boon of protein is its role in blood sugar regulation. Unlike other macronutrients, proteins cause a minimal rise in blood sugar levels. This gentle nudge to your insulin means you're less likely to experience the peaks and valleys that can lead to cravings and crashes. It's all about stable energy, keeping you satiated and sharp, and preventing those sneaky weight gain culprits from sabotaging your progress.

And if you're thinking about going plant-based or you're a vegetarian, no sweat – plant proteins can be just as effective. The key is combining different plant sources to ensure you get all the essential amino acids. Foods like quinoa, buckwheat, and soy are complete proteins on their own, while beans, nuts, and whole grains can be paired up for a full complement of amino acids. Get creative with combinations to make your plant-based diet a metabolism-boosting powerhouse.

What about protein shakes and bars, you ask? They're convenient, sure, but they should complement, not replace, whole food sources of protein. Whole foods come with additional nutrients that work synergistically to promote metabolic health. Use the supplements wisely and as part of an overall balanced diet, especially when whole foods aren't an option.

Let's not forget the synergy between protein intake and exercise. Imagine the dynamic duo of Batman and Robin, except it's protein and exercise fighting the crime of a sluggish metabolism. Protein helps repair and build muscle tissue, which is especially important after strength training exercises that create tiny tears in your muscles. With adequate protein, your body can repair and build stronger muscles – which, as noted earlier, are fantastically efficient calorie burners.

In conclusion, thinking of protein as just another nutrient underestimates its mighty role in resetting your metabolism. It's about eating smarter, not necessarily more – and this savvy approach to protein will contribute significantly to tipping the scales in your favor for weight loss. Keep the quality high, and the variety wide, and you'll be setting the stage for a metabolic makeover that fuels your weight loss journey, keeps you satisfied, and cruises past those plateaus with confidence.

The Importance of Micronutrients

As we hone in on nutrition's role in metabolism, it's critical to zoom in on the unsung heroes often eclipsed by their macronutrient counterparts: micronutrients. These minute compounds, required in smaller quantities, are mighty players in the metabolic game—one that's not just about weight loss, but fundamentally about achieving optimal health.

Don't let the "micro" prefix fool you; vitamins and minerals clock in some serious work. These nutrients facilitate countless biochemical reactions integral to metabolizing carbs, fats, and proteins into usable energy. For instance, B vitamins are like a high-end office manager that keeps energy production within the body running smoothly, coordinating the conversion of food into fuel your cells can expend.

Then there's the dynamic duo of iron and zinc, pivotal for their enzyme-assisting roles. Iron, central to transporting oxygen within the bloodstream, quite literally breathes life into metabolic processes, while zinc acts as a linchpin for over a hundred enzymatic reactions. Without them, your metabolic pathways would slow down, similar to a roadblock on a busy highway—troublesome, especially when you're aiming to fire up your metabolism.

Also playing a part in this nutritional ensemble are antioxidants, like vitamins C and E, and selenium. These substances help combat oxidative stress, a ceaseless battle within our bodies that can impede metabolic efficiency and play a role in weight management challenges. Imagine your metabolism as an energy-efficient engine; antioxidants help keep it clean and less prone to wear and tear, so it runs at peak performance.

Calcium and vitamin D also can't escape our attention given their role in maintaining a hearty skeleton. But their prowess extends beyond bone health. Did you know vitamin D receptors are found in nearly all body cells? Its presence suggests a wider influence—including on metabolic pathways—while calcium is crucial not just for bone integrity but also for aiding in the smooth execution of nerve transmission and muscle function.

What's more, micronutrients influence your metabolic speed indirectly by impacting your immune system. A resilient immune system is a pillar of good health, allowing you to maintain an active lifestyle which in turn supports a hearty metabolism. Without adequate micronutrient intake, your immunity may falter, leaving you sidelined, and consequently, slowing your metabolic rate.

Hydration and electrolyte balance, too, pivot on micronutrients. Minerals like potassium, sodium, and magnesium maintain fluid balance inside and outside of cells and a disturbance in this balance can lead to sluggish metabolic activity. Imagine an Olympic-sized pool: to swim efficiently, the water level must be just right; similarly, our cells require a precise balance of fluids and nutrients to function at their best.

Considering all these roles, it's clear that micronutrient deficiencies can throw a wrench into your metabolic efficiency. But how do you ensure you're getting enough? Eating a colorful array of fruits and vegetables, lean proteins, whole grains, and dairy can deliver a diverse cast of these microscopic stars. It's all about variety and balance—no one food group can provide all, but together, they make up a powerhouse supporting your metabolic health.

It's tempting to think popping a multivitamin could cover any dietary gaps. But while supplements can be beneficial, especially in cases of deficiencies, the body is better equipped to use nutrients derived from whole food sources. Think of it as preferring a live orchestra over a recorded tune—the experience and benefits are richer.

In the end, micronutrients may not be the lead singer on the nutrition stage, but without them, the band can't play. Supporting your metabolic rate is a complex affair that goes beyond just cutting calories and embracing macro ratios. Integrating a spectrum of vitamins and minerals is like assembling a top-notch team—each 'player' enhances the group's performance, leading to a metabolism that's fine-tuned for weight loss success and overall well-being.

Hydration and Metabolic Function

While carbs, fats, and proteins grab the nutritional spotlight, let's shift our focus to the unsung hero of metabolic function: water. This clear, calorie-free substance might seem passive, but it's actually a powerhouse when it comes to your metabolism. Imagine water as the oil in the engine of a car; without it, the machinery would overheat and grind to a halt. In the same way, your body needs adequate hydration to keep the metabolic gears running smoothly.

Your cells are mini-factories that perform metabolic reactions, and they need an aqueous environment to do so effectively. These processes include everything from breaking down food for energy to synthesizing hormones. Water does not merely provide the environment; it participates in these biochemical reactions. For example, it plays a crucial role in hydrolysis which splits molecules to release energy.

Think about the last time you felt dehydrated. That sluggish feeling wasn't just discomfort – it was a sign that your metabolic processes were not firing on all cylinders. Staying hydrated boosts your body's ability to burn calories efficiently. It has been shown that drinking water can temporarily spike metabolism by thermogenesis, meaning that your body uses energy to warm the water to body temperature, thus burning a few extra calories in the process.

Additionally, hydration has a direct effect on your liver functions, which plays a central role in converting fats to energy. Without enough water, your liver has to work harder, and fat metabolism becomes less efficient. This can slow down any weight loss efforts. Drinking plenty of fluids is essential to keep the liver and your metabolism humming.

Let's not forget the kinship between hydration and digestive health. Proper hydration ensures that your digestive system can move waste efficiently. When you're dehydrated, your body is more likely to experience constipation, which can make you feel bloated and could potentially interfere with the absorption of nutrients necessary for a healthy metabolism.

Furthermore, sipping water throughout the day can also lead to a decreased appetite. It's not unusual to confuse thirst with hunger, leading to overeating. Having a glass of water before meals can make you feel fuller, thus reducing the likelihood of consuming excess calories that your body might store as fat.

In the pursuit of resetting your metabolism, it's essential to remember that while water doesn't contain magical fat-burning properties, it does facilitate every metabolic process in your body. Balance is vital; too much water can lead to dilution of electrolytes, while too little can cause dehydration - both can upset your metabolic balance. So what's the magic number? You've likely heard the old adage of eight glasses a day, but the truth is, individual hydration needs vary. Factors include your physical activity level, the climate you live in, and your overall health.

To ensure you're getting enough but not overdoing it, listen to your body. Thirst is an obvious indicator, but also pay attention to the color of your urine - a light yellow means you're usually well-hydrated. It's not complicated; just like your metabolism, your body is smart, and it will tell you what it needs if you're willing to listen.

So, as you work to reset your metabolism and perhaps lose some weight, don't underestimate the impact that plain old water could have on your journey. It's calorie-free, generally available, and might just be the key to unlocking a more efficient metabolic rate. Keep a bottle or glass of water at your side and make hydration a priority in your daily routine. After all, fueling your metabolic fire requires the right balance of nutrients, and water is among the most crucial.

Now that we've drenched ourselves in the importance of hydration for metabolic function, remember it's only a piece of the puzzle. Pairing proper hydration with balanced nutrition and other lifestyle factors creates a synergy that can optimize your metabolism and support your weight loss efforts more effectively than any single component alone.

DAVID ALEXANDER

Chapter 5

The Power of Intermittent Fasting

As we turn the page on nutrition's direct impacts, we step into the fascinating realm of intermittent fasting and its substantial role in revamping your metabolism. This time-tested approach isn't just a fleeting trend; it's a lifestyle adjustment that draws on our evolutionary backstory, giving your body the pause it needs to optimize the weight loss process. Now, you might be thinking, how exactly does taking a break from eating fuel such profound changes? Imagine giving your digestive system its own mini-vacation, allowing it to reboot and engage in some much-needed cellular housekeeping. That's the magic of intermittent fasting! It empowers your hormones to dance to a tune that supports fat burn and urges your cells to renew and repair, setting the stage for a metabolism that functions with the ferocity and precision of a brand-new engine. And the best part? It's all hinged on timing—no need to overhaul your diet or subscribe to draconian eating habits. Strap in; we're about to embark on an exploration of how intermittent fasting can bridge the gap between where you stand today and where your metabolism thrives, fully ignited.

What Is Intermittent Fasting?

Picture this: a strategy so straightforward yet so effective that it can kick your metabolism into high gear without the need for complex dietary concoctions or over-the-top workout regimens. That strategy is intermittent fasting, a pattern of eating that alternates between periods of fasting and eating. It's not so much about what you eat, but when you eat it. This time-restricted approach to nourishment has been gathering applause for its potential to reset and revitalize the body's metabolic processes.

Intermittent fasting isn't a novel concept; in fact, it's been around since ancient times. Our ancestors often went without food for extended periods – not out of choice, but necessity – and it turns out, their bodies were well-equipped for these fasts. In the modern world, however, the abundance and accessibility of food have shifted us away from this intermittent eating pattern, potentially to the detriment of our metabolic health.

So, how exactly does intermittent fasting work? It taps into the body's innate ability to switch energy sources. When we eat, glucose is readily available and preferred for energy. However, during a fast, our glucose stores run low, prompting the body to burn stored fat for fuel. This metabolic switch is where the magic happens, improving insulin sensitivity and offering a host of potential health benefits.

What's fascinating is intermittent fasting's versatility. It can be adapted to fit almost any lifestyle or preference, with various fasting windows that make the practice achievable and sustainable. Whether it's the popular 16/8 method, with 16 hours of fasting followed by an 8-hour eating window, or alternate-day fasting, there's likely a method that can harmonize with your daily routine.

Intermittent fasting isn't a silver bullet, though - getting the timing right is crucial. It's about letting your body feast, and then taking a break long enough to trigger the processes responsible for the metabolic reset. It's not about starvation; it's about strategic timing to harness your body's biological rhythms in your favor.

One of the alluring aspects of intermittent fasting is its simplicity. There's no need to embark on a major diet overhaul or adhere to a rigid eating schedule. Instead, it's a reorganization of your existing patterns, providing a structure that promotes better health without the need for counting calories or macronutrient obsession.

But it's essential to enter intermittent fasting with a degree of caution and knowledge. It isn't suitable for everyone, and certain medical conditions or lifestyles may complicate its implementation. Moreover, the transition can come with side effects as the body adapts to new eating patterns. That's why it's vital to be informed and, when necessary, consult a healthcare professional.

Intermittent fasting's power lies in its potential to reshape the way your body handles energy, stimulates fat loss, and paves the way towards better overall health. With a resurgence of interest in the scientific community and glowing endorsements from those who've seen tangible results, it's a phenomenon that's hard to ignore.

For many, this flexible approach to eating could be the missing link in their health and weight loss endeavors. As you embark on this journey, remember that intermittent fasting isn't merely a diet; it's a lifestyle shift that, when incorporated sensibly, can lead to profound changes in your metabolic health.

We'll explore the different methods, delve into the biological benefits, and weigh the precautions in the following sections. For now, immerse yourself in the concept of intermittent fasting as a potent lever to reset your body's natural rhythms, paving the way for weight loss and metabolic rejuvenation.

Different Methods of Intermittent Fasting

As we dive deeper into the transformative world of intermittent fasting (IF), it's crucial to understand that there isn't a one-size-fits-all approach. Varied IF methods cater to different lifestyles, preferences, and goals. Whether you're a busy parent juggling work and kids, or someone looking for an edge in metabolic health, there's a style that fits your life like a key in a lock.

First up is the popular **16/8 method**, also known as the Lean Gains protocol, which involves fasting for a 16-hour window and eating during an 8-hour window each day. Many find this to be a sustainable approach as it can be as simple as skipping breakfast and making lunch your first meal. Imagine firing up your metabolism daily while still enjoying a hearty dinner every evening.

Then there's the **5:2 diet**, where you eat normally for five days a week and restrict calories to about 500-600 for the other two non-consecutive days. This method allows for regular eating patterns most days, which can be mentally less daunting for those new to IF.

For those who love a challenge, the **eat-stop-eat** strategy might be captivating. This involves a full 24-hour fast once or twice a week. It's a test of willpower, true, but the sense of achievement after conquering a full day without food can be as sweet as the first bite into your post-fast meal.

If daily fasting feels overwhelming, the **alternate day fasting** could be more your speed. This protocol alternates between days of normal eating and days of either complete fasting or limited calorie intake. It's a rhythm that dances to the beat of a different drum, providing flexibility and a challenge.

For the morning enthusiasts, there's the **Warrior Diet**. This format features 20 hours of fasting with a 4-hour eating window at night, focusing on small portions of raw fruits and vegetables during the day and one large meal in the evening. It's based on the eating patterns of ancient warriors, who, legend has it, had a robust metabolism to match their strength.

Another variant is the **12-hour fast**, which, as the name suggests, splits the day evenly between fasting and eating. It's a gentle introduction to the world of IF, making it less intimidating for beginners. Ease into fasting without feeling like you're taking the deep plunge right away.

Modification of these methods is also possible, like the **14/10 method** — a slight relaxation of the 16/8 protocol for those finding a 16-hour fast too stringent. It's all about making IF work for you, not twisting your life to meet its demands.

The beauty of IF lies in its versatility. You can always start with one method and switch to another if the first doesn't quite mesh with your daily routine. What's more, you can adjust your eating window on specific days based on your social life or work demands. The goal isn't to imprison your lifestyle; it's to liberate your metabolism. So, it's essential to be flexible and forgiving as you find the rhythm that works for you.

Remember that while the methodology may vary, the core philosophy of intermittent fasting remains the same: cycle between periods of fasting and eating to reset and revitalize your metabolism. Each method has its unique perks and challenges, and there's a certain thrill in finding the one that clicks with you—a dance between discipline and freedom, structure, and flexibility.

Finally, consistency is king. Whether you choose to fast for part of the day or part of the week, what matters most is sticking with it. Your body's metabolism doesn't shift overnight, but give it time, and it can adapt to this new pattern of eating, potentially unlocking a refreshed, more vibrant version of you.

Benefits and Cautions

As we've explored intermittent fasting (IF) and its role in metabolic reset, it's time to weigh the benefits against the potential risks, ensuring an informed and safe approach to this lifestyle change. The concept of IF isn't just a fleeting trend; its roots are grounded in evidence-based research, showing a bounty of health gains when executed correctly.

Starting with the positives, IF can be incredibly powerful in resetting your metabolism. By cycling between periods of eating and fasting, your body learns to utilize fat stores for energy, leading to weight loss without the need for calorie counting or obsessive meal tracking. This process not only trims your waistline but also sharpens mental clarity, with studies noting increased cognitive function during fasting states.

Furthermore, IF can improve insulin sensitivity, which is crucial for those grappling with prediabetic conditions or type 2 diabetes. When your insulin levels are well-managed, you're less likely to experience the energy dips and cravings that can derail your diet plans. There's also a boost in growth hormone production, aiding in muscle preservation and potentially en-hancing longevity.

Yet, for all its perks, IF isn't without its caveats. It's essential to recog-nize that this approach isn't one-size-fits-all. While some thrive on a 16:8 regimen, others may find 24-hour fasts more beneficial. In this personal journey, listening to your body's signals is key to avoiding adverse effects.

And cautions do exist. Those with a history of eating disorders should steer clear of IF, as it could potentially trigger unhealthy behaviors or thought patterns. Additionally, women, especially those trying to conceive, preg-nant, or breastfeeding, should consult with a healthcare provider before starting IF due to its potential impact on reproductive hormones.

Another note of caution regards training. While some find that their workouts are not hampered by fasting, others may experience decreased performance or recovery issues. It's vital to adjust your exercise intensity and timing to mesh seamlessly with your fasting schedule.

Hydration and nutrient intake can't be ignored either. During eating win-dows, it's crucial to focus on nutrient-dense foods to compensate for the extended periods without nourishment. Falling into the trap of consum-ing high-calorie, low-nutrient foods can negate the benefits of IF, leading to potential nutritional deficiencies and a lack of energy.

Moreover, IF isn't a miracle cure. It doesn't give carte blanche to disregard other aspects of health, like sleep quality, stress management, and overall diet quality, all of which play a central role in metabolic health. And on that note, IF should be viewed as a component of a holistic lifestyle change—one that encompasses a balanced diet, regular physical activity, and adequate rest.

It's also wise to introduce IF gradually. Jumping straight into a rigorous fasting regimen can be a shock to the system, potentially causing headaches, lethargy, and irritability. Start slow, allowing your body to acclimate to this new pattern of eating.

Considering these benefits and cautions, the key takeaway is that although IF can be a robust tool for metabolic reset, it requires a nuanced and personalized approach. Listen to your body, do your research, and if necessary, collaborate with a health professional to ensure that you're embarking on this journey safely and effectively.

Chapter 6

Detox Your Body for Metabolic Success

Stepping into the realm of detoxification can spark a transformative stage in your metabolic reset journey. A well-implemented detox is like giving your body a refreshing cleanse, ridding it of the toxins that could be bogging down your metabolism. But let's clear the air first—detoxing isn't about harsh fasts or extreme cleanses. It's about fine-tuning your body's natural cleaning systems for optimal metabolic performance.

Fascination with detoxification has taken society by storm, with trendy juices and fasting regimes making headlines. However, it's not as complex as it's made out to be. Your body already has a sophisticated detox system in place, courtesy of your liver, kidneys, digestive system, and even your skin. But, the trick lies in optimizing these systems' efficiency through lifestyle and dietary choices for better metabolic function.

What Does Detox Mean?

When we dive into the process of enhancing our metabolic success, the term 'detox' invariably swims into view. But let's clear the waters right away: detox isn't about drastic cleanses or the extreme restriction of food groups. No, it's about giving our bodies a breather—a chance to recalibrate and dispose of the burdens that may be slowing us down.

Detoxification, fundamentally, is our body's multifaceted system of cleansing itself from the inside out. Our liver works around the clock, filtering through the good, the bad, and the downright unhealthy substances we consume. This isn't just about alcohol or processed food; even the air we breathe can bring in toxins that need processing. But sometimes, the load becomes a bit too much, and our bodies signal for some maintenance.

A proper detox focuses on supporting our natural systems, particularly the liver, kidneys, and digestive system, ensuring they can do their jobs effectively. It's not the mythical purge that often gets sold to us in glitzy marketing campaigns. Instead, it's about creating an internal environment conducive to optimal metabolic function—aptly akin to tidying up your living space for clarity and efficiency.

Think of balancing your body like you would a well-kept garden. Just as you'd weed out invasive plants and nourish the soil, detoxing eliminates foods and habits that hinder metabolic health while fortifying your body with what it truly needs to thrive. It's about mindfully curating your intake to support detoxification pathways, championing whole foods, hydration, and nutrients over processed sugar-laden temptations.

Now, don't expect overnight miracles. Detoxification is an ongoing process, not a one-off event. It's about integrating practices that support your body's natural rhythms and giving it the ongoing care it deserves. This could mean choosing organic produce to lessen the load of pesticides, sipping on water infused with fresh lemon to provide a gentle liver flush, or savoring cruciferous vegetables that ramp up detox enzymes.

Embracing a detox mindset isn't about depriving yourself; it's about mindful indulgence in what benefits you most. Opting for green tea over soda does more than cut down sugar—it inundates your system with antioxidants. Savoring fatty fish grants you omega-3 fatty acids, crucial for dampening inflammation which can otherwise contribute to metabolic sluggishness.

Let's not forget—detox is also about what we don't put into our bodies. Steering clear of toxins such as tobacco smoke, limiting alcohol intake, and curbing exposure to environmental pollutants like poor air quality play a significant role in our metabolic reset. By reducing these burdens, we facilitate our body's natural detox processes, giving our metabolism the upper hand.

Of course, it would be remiss to ignore movement as a detox ally. Sweat isn't just a sign of a good workout; it's your body's way of expelling toxins. Regular physical activity enhances blood flow, which in turn optimizes toxin elimination, not to mention the myriad of benefits it brings to metabolic health.

At its core, a detox is about giving your body the respect and attention it needs for peak performance. Counter to the quick-fix stories with which we're often bombarded, real detoxification is subtle and grounded in everyday choices. Our bodies are equipped with remarkable systems designed to keep us balanced; sometimes, they just need a bit of assistance. Detox, in essence, means committing to the choices that will enable these systems to run smoothly, ensuring that we pave the way for metabolic success.

So, as you contemplate starting on a path to reset your metabolism, consider detox not as a fad or a temporary fix, but as a sustainable practice—a vital part of your lifestyle that underpins the robust functioning of your internal systems. Consider this chapter a starting block for uncovering the secrets of detoxing done right, setting the stage for an environment where your metabolism doesn't just survive; it thrives.

Safe and Effective Detox Strategies

Embarking on a journey to reset your metabolism isn't just about what you feed your body, but also about how you cleanse it. Detox strategies have gained immense popularity and, although they're often misunderstood, they can be super instruments for paving the way to metabolic success. Remember, detoxification is about supporting your body's natural systems for filtering out the unwanted guests—think toxins and waste products—and a safe detox goes hand in hand with boosting your metabolic efficiency.

First things first, hydrate. I can't stress enough the magic that is water—nature's elixir. Ensuring you're well-hydrated aids your kidneys and liver, the star players in detoxification. But it isn't just about the quantity; the quality of the water matters too. Opt for filtered water when possible, and kickstart your day with a warm lemon water drink to stimulate your digestive system.

Next on the list is your diet. A detox-friendly diet is rich in whole foods like leafy greens, berries, and nuts. These foods are loaded with antioxidants, fiber, vitamins, and minerals that bolster your body's detox systems. A common misconception is that you need to restrict calories to detox effectively, but it's really about being mindful of what you eat. Include cruciferous vegetables, like broccoli and Brussels sprouts, which contain compounds that help regulate detox enzymes in the liver.

Another key strategy is leveraging the power of herbs and spices. Today, let's spotlight turmeric with its active compound curcumin, revered for its anti-inflammatory and liver-detoxifying properties. Adding turmeric to your meals or sipping on a turmeric-laced tea could do wonders for your detoxification pathways.

Let's not forget about certainly one of your body's natural detoxifiers—sweat. Regular exercise not only ramps up your metabolism but also promotes sweating, which helps expel toxins through your skin. Whether it's a brisk walk or a high-intensity gym session, getting your heart pumping is a win for your overall health.

Speaking of exercise, have you considered the calming waves of yoga to bolster your detox efforts? Yoga poses like twists can massage internal organs, promoting the elimination of toxins. Plus, the focused breathing is like a broom, sweeping away the cobwebs of stress, which can often hinder your body's detox abilities.

Let's talk about the environments where we spend most of our time—our homes. Detoxing isn't merely about what you ingest or how you move; it's also ensuring your living space isn't contributing to your body's toxin load. Use natural cleaning products, and be wary of plastics and other materials that can leach chemicals into your food and skin.

Detox doesn't equal deprivation. An effective detox plan should leave you feeling nourished, not starved. Space out your meals and aim for balanced portions; this helps your digestive system process foods more efficiently, ensuring the optimum absorption of nutrients needed for detoxification.

For those considering fasting as a detox method, it's essential to approach it with caution and knowledge. While intermittent fasting can support detoxification by giving your digestive system a rest, extreme fasting or "cleanses" can backfire. Always listen to your body, and consider seeking advice from a healthcare provider before embarking on a fasting journey.

Last but not least, let's focus on rest. Sleep is an often underestimated detoxifier. During sleep, your brain actively removes toxins that have accumulated throughout the day through a process known as the glymphatic system. Quality sleep not only supports this process but also helps regulate the hormones that influence your metabolism.

Implementing safe and effective detox strategies can be a fulfilling part of your metabolic reset. Each step you take contributes to a cleaner, more efficient body that's primed for metabolic success. As you incorporate these practices into your life, you'll likely find your energy levels rising, your skin glowing, and that sluggish metabolism turning into a dynamic engine propelling you forward in your health journey.

Foods to Support Detoxification

Taking a step from understanding the overarching theme of detoxification, it's about time we zoomed in on specific foods that will be your allies in this journey. When you're resetting your metabolism, nourishing your body with the right foods is like hitting the refresh button—essential, invigorating, and downright transformative. So, let's get down to the brass tacks and lay out the kind of grub that's going to support your body's natural detoxification processes.

Ever heard of *cruciferous vegetables*? Broccoli, cauliflower, Brussels sprouts, and their family members are more than just side dishes. They're packed with compounds like sulforaphane which not only give them their slightly bitter edge, but also support the liver enzymes in the detox process. These heavy lifters don't just go through the motions; they actively help in eliminating toxins and free radicals that can slow your metabolic fire.

We can't talk detox without giving a nod to the green giant—*leafy greens*. Kale, spinach, and chard are not just trendy; they're troves of chlorophyll which binds to toxins and helps clear them out. They're the vacuums of the vegetable world if you will, that help your body purge the pesky toxins hiding in the nooks and crannies of your cells.

Next up, meet your detox dream team players: *garlic* and *onions*. These pungent powerhouses are loaded with sulfur-containing compounds that take the reins in detoxifying the body. They're naturals at fighting off harmful invaders and making sure your metabolic engine is purring smoothly. Try them sautéed, roasted, or raw if you can handle the kick—they're versatile enough to perk up any dish and your detox efforts.

You've likely been told an apple a day keeps the doctor away, but did you know this crisp treat is also a detox delight? Pectin, a type of soluble fiber found in *apples*, is like a sponge in the digestive tract, soaking up toxins and helping expel them from the body. Plus, they're a sweet source of antioxidants that can rev up your metabolic rate to boot.

Let's not forget about the understated, yet mighty *beets*. With their deep crimson hue, they're not just for staining cutting boards; they're brimming with natural plant compounds that reinforce detoxification enzymes in the liver. Syncing up with the body's detox pathways, beets are essentially a clean-up crew for your blood, ensuring toxins are not just shuffled around, but actually shown the exit.

Remember to soak up some lemony sunshine too. A squeeze of *lemon* in your water isn't just for flavor—it's a simple and refreshing way to encourage your liver to do a little extra heavy lifting in the detox department. High in vitamin C, lemons offer more than a tangy taste; they bring on board their antioxidant prowess, battling potential toxins and aiding in their removal.

Imagine your body is like a complex machine, and these foods are the premium oil that keeps it running smoothly. An oil change is sometimes all you need to get back into gear, and incorporating these detox-supporting foods into your diet is akin to that—revitalizing and necessary. Your metabolism's efficiency can be substantially influenced by the quality of what you put into it.

Lastly, remember hydration. The clear, tasteless liquid that flows from your taps – *water*. Hydration facilitates the transport of nutrients and removal of waste, and simply put, without it, your body can't detox properly. Water sets the stage for every biochemical reaction in the body, including those that power up your metabolism and those that clean shop.

To wrap it up, stacking your diet with these detox-friendly foods isn't just about dropping weight; it's about giving your body the respect and care it deserves. It's about supporting your body's innate cleaning system so it can do what it's designed to do—only better. So, enrich your meals with these nutritious champs and watch as your metabolism thanks you with the vigor and vitality you need to conquer each day.

Hang around for what's next because this is just the starting line. We will dive deeper into the ocean of metabolic mysteries in the following sections and chapters, ensuring you're fully equipped to take on your metabolic success with confidence and clarity.

Chapter 7

Balancing Your Blood Sugar

As we peel back another layer of the metabolic mystique, it's time to zero in on a cornerstone of metabolic control: blood sugar balance. Ever wonder why you're raided by relentless cravings, or why your energy seems to nosedive without warning? It could all come down to the rollercoaster ride your blood sugar levels are taking you on—and getting off that ride is crucial to resetting your metabolism and tipping the scales in your favor. Imagine your body as a finely tuned machine; it needs the right kind of fuel at the right times to run smoothly. This isn't about depriving yourself or adhering to extreme diets; it's about smart, sustainable practices that maintain a steady stream of energy to your cells. So let's get into the nitty-gritty, the science-backed strategies that will help you achieve that elusive balance, and set the stage for weight loss that sticks. By taming your blood sugar, you can temper your appetite, bolster your energy, and fire up your metabolism—let's embark on this transformative journey together.

Blood Sugar Regulation and Metabolism

You've probably heard that maintaining balanced blood sugar levels is crucial for good health, but have you ever wondered why? The body's ability to regulate blood sugar is a linchpin in our metabolic processes. It's much more than just avoiding the highs and lows that can make you feel like you're on an emotional and physical roller coaster. It's about creating a stable environment where weight loss isn't just possible—it's probable.

At its core, blood sugar regulation involves two key players: insulin and glucagon. These hormones work in a tight partnership to maintain blood glucose levels within a narrow range. Insulin, often described as a 'storage hormone,' helps cells absorb glucose, reducing blood sugar levels, and signaling the body to store fat. Conversely, glucagon tells the liver to release stored glucose when blood sugar drops, ensuring you have energy between meals. The stability of this give-and-take is what keeps us on an even keel, metabolically speaking.

Now, here's the kicker: when we consistently overload our system with simple carbs and sugars, this system starts to break down. Insulin keeps being released in high amounts, leading eventually to cells becoming less responsive to it—a state called insulin resistance. This can be the beginning of a cascade of metabolic problems, starting with weight gain and potentially leading to conditions like type 2 diabetes.

Let's consider the analogy of a locked door. If insulin is the key, and the cell is the locked door, resistance is like changing the locks. Eventually, the key doesn't fit, and glucose stays in the bloodstream. Now, you're dealing with high blood sugar levels and a reduced ability to burn fat because your cells can't get the energy they need.

So, what's to be done? Managing your macro intake can be a game changer. Complex carbohydrates, rich in fiber, don't spike your blood sugar the way simple sugars do. They take longer to break down, providing a more controlled release of energy and keeping insulin levels stable. This slow-burning energy is what we're after, as it encourages the body to convert stored fat to fuel rather than constantly dealing with new influxes of sugars.

Regular, balanced meals play a huge role in this process. When we skip meals, we risk letting our blood glucose drop too low and subsequently rebound with intense cravings for quick sugars. This can lead to a cycle of spikes and crashes that wreak havoc on our metabolism. Rather than skipping meals, focusing on a balanced diet rich in fibers, healthy fats, and lean proteins can foster a steady supply of energy and balance our blood sugar levels.

Exercise is also a potent tool. Physical activity increases insulin sensitivity, which means that cells are better able to use available insulin to absorb glucose during and after activity. In essence, exercise is like a lubricant for that lock and key mechanism we talked about earlier—it keeps everything working smoothly.

Now, all this talk about balanced meals and exercise is fine and dandy, but there's something else that often flies under the radar: stress. Chronic stress can lead to high levels of cortisol, a hormone that can increase blood sugar levels. Learning to manage stress through practices such as mindfulness, meditation, or even just taking a daily walk can have significant benefits for blood sugar regulation.

And don't forget about sleep! When we're sleep-deprived, the body craves energy, and unfortunately, sugar and simple carbs seem like the quickest solution. Ensure you're getting the recommended 7-9 hours of sleep per night to aid in regulating hormones and maintaining blood sugar levels.

Ultimately, taking control of blood sugar regulation is an empowering step towards a healthier metabolism. It's not an overnight process, but by consistently making mindful choices about diet and lifestyle, you're setting the stage for sustained weight loss and overall better health. Listen to your body and give it the support it needs—your metabolism will thank you for it.

Strategies for Maintaining Stable Blood Sugar Levels

Let's dive into the beating heart of stable metabolism—keeping those blood sugar levels steady. With the immediacy of modern life, it can be all too easy to let regular eating habits slide, only to be hit by waves of fatigue or hunger pangs. But here's the thing: by stabilizing your blood sugar, you're not only supporting your metabolism but also setting the stage for sustained weight loss success. Let's go through some practical strategies that make a difference.

First and foremost, favor **fiber-rich foods**. We're talking fruits, vegetables, legumes, and whole grains. Fiber slows down glucose absorption into your bloodstream, minimizing those pesky spikes. Switch out white bread for whole grain, and snack on a handful of berries instead of that candy bar. Simple swaps can yield real results in your blood sugar levels.

Another key component is **protein**. Incorporating a decent serving of protein in every meal can help balance blood sugar by providing a steady energy source. It can also curb hunger, preventing overeating. Whether it's chicken, tofu, or a scoop of almond butter, these additions can make your meals more balanced and help sidestep those sudden sugar crashes.

And let's not overlook the importance of **healthy fats**. Avocados, nuts, and seeds contain fats that help moderate blood sugar and keep you feeling full longer. Instead of reaching for a low-fat option that might be packed with sugars, choose the full-fat version—it's likely to do you more favors in the blood sugar department.

Timing is crucial as well. Eating smaller, more frequent meals can prevent the rollercoaster effect that can come from waiting too long to eat and then binging. Grab a small, balanced snack between meals to keep your metabolism ticking over and to stay ahead of hunger.

What about when you've got that sweet tooth? Opt for natural sweeteners like **stevia or monk fruit**, which don't spike your glucose levels the way refined sugars do. But always remember, moderation is key—even natural sweeteners can disrupt your balanced eating pattern if overused.

Don't forget to stay **hydrated**. Drinking enough water is often overlooked when talking about blood sugar, but it assists in filtering out excess glucose through the kidneys. And quite often, what we mistake for hunger may actually be thirst in disguise.

Moving beyond dietary tweaks, regular **physical activity** is a powerhouse for maintaining stable blood sugar levels. Exercise pulls glucose from your blood for energy, naturally lowering levels. Think of your muscles as sponges that soak up that glucose right out of your bloodstream, whether it's through a brisk walk, sprint, or lifting some weights.

What about those nights out or celebrations? Here's a golden rule: Don't arrive famished. Have a balanced snack before you go; it'll help you avoid diving headfirst into high-sugar temptations. Also, by savoring your meal and eating slowly, you give your body the chance to maintain a balanced sugar level as you digest.

Lastly, understand that maintaining stable blood sugar is a daily commitment, but also a matter of balance and consistency. Sticking to a routine that includes a mix of fiber, protein, and healthy fats will do wonders for keeping your blood sugar even-keeled. Pair that with regular movement and hydration, and you're well on your way to metabolic success.

As you incorporate these strategies into your daily regime, you'll notice less hunger fluctuations, and a more engaged and energetic self, and yes—the scale might start tipping in your favor. Just remember, resetting your metabolism is a game of strategic placement. Every choice you make either adds a steadying piece to your metabolic puzzle or takes one away—choose wisely.

Chapter 8

The Gut-Metabolism Connection

As we dive deeper into the journey of resetting our metabolism, let's not overlook the bustling metropolis that is our digestive system. It's about time we got up close and personal with the gut-metabolism axis—a crucial player in the weight management game. Think of your gut as a garden; what you plant, how you tend to it, and the quality of the soil all impact what blossoms. Similarly, our gut flora, with its trillions of bacteria, profoundly influences how we process food, balance our blood glucose levels, and even dictate our cravings. Ever felt like your gut has a mind of its own? Well, in a way, it does. This chapter will unfold the mystery of how your gut health directly links to metabolic rate and energy usage, and we'll uncover how nurturing a healthy microbiome can be your secret weapon in shedding those stubborn pounds. We're not just feeding ourselves with every bite we take—we're feeding an entire ecosystem that, in return, can supercharge our metabolism. Don't worry; we'll sidestep any pseudoscientific nonsense and stick to real, actionable insights that can genuinely revamp your metabolic health. So, let's feed that inner garden with knowledge, fostering a symbiotic relationship that's poised to ignite your metabolic potential.

Understanding Gut Health

As we delve into the intertwined world of gut health and metabolism, it's important to grasp just how vital a well-functioning digestive system is to our overall well-being. The gut is not only a pathway for absorbing nutrients but also a complex ecosystem teeming with bacteria that play a pivotal role in how our bodies function, including the metabolic processes that govern our energy levels and weight.

Think of your gut as a bustling metropolis where trillions of microorganisms reside, each with specific roles that contribute to the city's overall operations. This microbiome is responsible for breaking down food, synthesizing vitamins, and even communicating with our brain through hormones and neural pathways. The diversity and balance of these microbial populations are critical to our health, influencing everything from digestion to immune function.

But what happens when this delicate ecosystem is disrupted? An imbalance, often referred to as dysbiosis, can lead to a cascade of health issues, including inflammation, obesity, and even chronic diseases. Your diet, lifestyle, stress levels, and antibiotic use are just a few factors that can impact the state of your gut health.

To maintain a healthy gut, it's paramount to eat a diet rich in varied and whole foods. Consuming fiber, found in fruits, vegetables, and whole grains, nurtures beneficial bacteria and supports the integrity of your gut lining. Additionally, reducing the intake of processed foods, which often contain emulsifiers and artificial sweeteners, is equally important, as these can disrupt your microbiome's harmony.

Let's not forget hydration – water is essential for nourishing gut mucosa and facilitating the smooth transit of digestible materials. Just as a city's plumbing system requires water to function properly, so does your digestive tract need adequate fluids to effectively transport waste and nutrients.

While it may go unnoticed, stress also wears on our gut health. Chronic stress can alter the gut's nervous system, causing a slew of digestive issues. This is why incorporating stress-reducing techniques like meditation, exercise, or simply ensuring adequate rest can be as crucial for your gut as it is for your mind.

Another key to supporting a healthy gut is nurturing the right kinds of bacteria. This is where probiotics enter the scene. These beneficial microorganisms can help restore balance to your gut flora, potentially easing digestive discomfort and contributing to a more robust metabolism. Fermented foods like yogurt, kefir, kombucha, and kimchi are natural sources of these friendly bacteria.

Inflammation is a term we often encounter, yet its impact on gut health is monumental. Chronic inflammation in the gut can lead to increased permeability of the intestinal lining, sometimes referred to as 'leaky gut'. This condition can agitate the immune system and contribute to metabolic dysregulation, laying the groundwork for weight gain and insulin resistance.

Lastly, it's crucial to account for individual differences when considering gut health. Factors like genetics and medication can influence the composition of the gut microbiome. Paying attention to how your body reacts to certain foods and adjusting your diet accordingly is an empowering step towards personalized gut health management.

In conclusion, nurturing our gut health is not just about dietary choices; it's about embracing a lifestyle that supports the entire ecosystem within us. By doing so, we create a favorable environment for our metabolic processes to thrive, ultimately supporting our weight loss goals and advancing our overall health. The gut is a remarkable ally in our health journey, and by understanding and caring for it, we set ourselves up for a lifetime of wellness.

Probiotics, Prebiotics, and Your Metabolism

As we've unraveled the complexities of gut health and its impact on overall well-being, we've stumbled upon some powerful allies in our quest for metabolic mastery: probiotics and prebiotics. These two players are the dynamic duo when it comes to nurturing a flourishing gut microbiome, and they hold the keys to potentially resetting and revving up your metabolism. But let's break down how these tiny titans work their magic from the inside out.

Probiotics, simply put, are live beneficial bacteria that you can ingest through certain foods or supplements. They're like friendly troops parachuting into the gut, taking residence, and contributing to a balanced microbiome. Why does this matter for your metabolism? Because a well-balanced gut flora has been linked to improved digestion, absorption of nutrients, and an enhanced immune response, all of which can positively influence your metabolic health.

Think of your gut as a garden. Just as plants need good soil and fertilizer to grow, so do these probiotic bacteria require nourishing substances to thrive. And that's where prebiotics come into play. Prebiotics are non-digestible fibers found in foods like chicory root, garlic, onions, and bananas.

They act as food for your gut's probiotics, helping them reproduce and maintain a strong fortification against harmful pathogens.

The synergistic effect of probiotics and prebiotics goes beyond just supporting a healthy gut environment; they directly interact with various metabolic pathways. For instance, some probiotic strains can impact our insulin sensitivity — a key player in the world of metabolism — and regulate hormones that signal hunger and fullness, affecting your body weight management.

Moreover, tweaking your intake of prebiotics and probiotics can modulate the gut-liver axis. This interaction influences how your body processes fats and balances sugar levels. And let's face it, who wouldn't want a finely tuned system that can fend off those pesky cravings and keep the energy levels steady?

However, it's not just about popping probiotic supplements like candy. Your digestive system craves variety. Incorporating a range of fermented foods into your diet, from yogurt to kimchi to sauerkraut, can introduce a diverse cast of bacterial strains. Diversity in your gut microbiome is akin to having a complete toolbox; it ensures your body can tackle multiple tasks efficiently, supporting a robust metabolism.

But here's the clincher: It's not enough to just add these microbe-friendly foods to your diet once in a blue moon. Consistency is key. Making prebiotics and probiotics a regular feature on your plate ensures their continued benefit to your gut community and, by extension, your metabolism. By feeding the good bacteria, you're essentially investing in the health of your digestive system and its ability to support a healthy weight.

Let's not forget, that the state of your gut can also impact how you feel day to day. Imbalances in gut bacteria are often associated with feelings of fatigue and sluggishness – symptoms that you don't need tagging along on your journey to metabolic renewal. By prioritizing gut health through probiotics and prebiotics, you're paving the way not just for a healthier metabolism, but also for a more vibrant, energetic you.

It's worth mentioning that the world of gut flora is highly individual. What works for one person's metabolism may not work for another's. This calls for a bit of trial and error and perhaps some professional guidance to pinpoint the perfect probiotic and prebiotic pairing for your unique system.

So, as part of your metabolic reset, take a closer look at your gut – it might just be the secret ingredient you've been missing in your recipe for weight loss success. By embracing the power of probiotics and prebiotics, you're not just facilitating weight loss; you're setting the stage for a lifetime of better health.

A Diet for a Healthy Gut

Transitioning from a focus on hormones and blood sugar regulation, let's zero in on your gut's well-being—a lesser-known but significant player in the metabolism game. You've probably heard the term' gut health' tossed around, but let's unpack what it truly means and, more importantly, how you nourish it with the right diet.

The gut, believe it or not, is your second brain, and there's a constant back-and-forth between what's going on in your stomach and what's going on with your metabolism. To keep this communication crisp and beneficial, you'll want to feed your gastrointestinal (GI) system foods that promote a balanced and diverse microbiome. So, what's on the menu for a healthy gut?

Let's start with *fiber*. We're talking fruits, vegetables, legumes, and whole grains—these are the deal-breakers of gut health. Fiber is the unsung hero that your body can't digest, but your beneficial gut bacteria thrive on it. It's like throwing a banquet for the good microbes, allowing them to multiply and, in turn, enhance your metabolic functioning.

Next up, we're looking at fermented foods. Think yogurt, kefir, sauerkraut, kombucha, and kimchi—these are not just trendy foods for the health-conscious. They're packed with probiotics, the friendly bacteria that you want to take up residence in your digestive tract. They can help balance your gut flora, which has a ripple effect on metabolic health.

Prebiotics shouldn't be overshadowed by their probiotic cousins. These are substances found in foods such as garlic, onions, bananas, and oatmeal that nourish the beneficial bacteria already in your gut. Together, prebiotics and probiotics work in tandem to ensure your digestive system is a well-oiled machine.

Diversity is key in a gut-healthy diet. A variety of plants in your diet can support a wide range of bacteria, each playing a different role in digestion and metabolism. Essentially, mix things up on your plate; an array of colors and types of food is not only visually appealing but beneficial for your insides, too.

But it's not just about what to add; it's also about what to limit. High-fat diets, especially those with unhealthy fats, and excessive sugar can throw your gut flora into a tailspin. Minimize processed foods—they're like a wrecking ball for your gut, causing inflammation and may hamper your metabolism.

Hydration is another pillar. Just like every other part of your body, your gut needs water to function at its best. Fluids help move fiber through your system and keep the mucosal lining of the gut in prime condition. So, don't skimp on those water breaks!

And what about food sensitivities? They're the thorn in your side, causing inflammation and disrupting gut harmony. Pay attention to how your body reacts to different foods. Consider eliminating culprits like gluten or lactose if they're not working in your favor.

Finally, timing matters. Eating regular meals and snacks can support a healthy gut rhythm. Long periods without food can disrupt your gut bacteria just as much as your blood sugar levels, so keep your eating schedule consistent.

It might seem like a lot to take in, but think of your dietary choices not just as a means to fuel your day but as messages to your microbiome, influencing everything from your mood to your metabolic rate. A gut-friendly diet is a cornerstone of overall health, and with each fiber-rich, probiotic-packed, and colorful meal, you're taking steps toward metabolic victory.

Just remember, there's no one-size-fits-all when it comes to your gut. It's all about finding the right balance for your body. With a diet that caters to a healthy gut, you're paving the way for a robust metabolism, better weight management, and an overall happier, healthier you.

Chapter 9

The Importance of Sleep in Metabolism

As we've delved into the intricate dance of hormones and gut health influencing your metabolism, it's time to turn off the lights and focus on a pillar of metabolic health just as critical – sleep! Trust me, when it comes to revving up your metabolism, catching those Z's is as important as the food on your plate or the weights you lift. It isn't just about quantity; quality matters too. Poor sleep can mess with your body's hunger hormones, leading to those late-night fridge raids that sabotage weight loss. And don't get me started on sleep's role in muscle recovery and blood sugar balance – crucial factors in a well-oiled metabolic machine. In this chapter, we'll dissect how sleep acts like a silent conductor of your metabolic orchestra, syncing up all the players for a harmonious performance. Grab your favorite pillow and get ready to dream your way to a leaner, meaner metabolism. Consider this your wake-up call (pun intended) – sleep isn't just a pause from daily hustle; it's prime time for metabolic magic. Let's unlock the nocturnal secrets that can set your metabolic reset on the right track!

How Sleep Affects Metabolism

If you've ever dragged through your day bleary-eyed and yawning, reaching for that third cup of coffee to stave off the sleepiness, you're likely aware that sleep can impact many facets of our lives. However, it's not just about feeling alert and focused; sleep plays a pivotal role in the behind-the-scenes action of our metabolism. In fact, skimping on sleep can seriously derail metabolic processes that are crucial for overall health and an effective metabolism.

When we slide into the arms of Morpheus, our body doesn't just switch off. Rather, it's a time of restoration and hormonal recalibration. One of the hormones taking the night shift is insulin, the gatekeeper that allows glucose to enter our cells. Poor sleep can lead to a less responsive insulin, which means sugar stays in the bloodstream longer, a condition known to us as insulin resistance. This can build a path towards weight gain, type 2 diabetes, and a slower metabolism. Getting adequate rest helps keep this hormone functioning properly.

Similarly, ghrelin and leptin, our hunger hormones, are influenced by our sleep habits. Ghrelin tells us when we're hungry, and leptin gives the signal to put down the fork. However, when we don't catch enough zzz's, ghrelin levels spike. At the same time, leptin takes a nosedive, which means you're more likely to indulge in that late-night snack or overeat the next day.

We also can't ignore the role of growth hormone, which is predominantly released during deep sleep. This hormone isn't just about getting taller; it's essential for muscle repair, building lean mass, and thus stoking the metabolic furnace that burns calories even when we're at rest. Restrictive sleep could be cutting into your body's natural anabolic processes.

Moreover, lack of sleep tends to promote inflammation and oxidative stress, both of which are sworn enemies of a healthy metabolism. They can impair the way your body processes and stores energy, leading to a sluggish metabolic rate, which can throw a wrench in your weight loss goals.

But it's not just about a single night of bad sleep. It's the chronic, tossing-and-turning, consistently poor-quality sleep patterns that can really add up. Over time, the effects of sleep deprivation compound like interest in a savings account, except what you're accumulating is metabolic debt. Each restless night is like a withdrawal from your metabolic health account, one that can grow over time and become harder to pay back.

Consider also cortisol, the stress hormone that tells your body to conserve energy to fuel your waking hours. Chronically high levels of cortisol, often a product of inadequate sleep, will signal your body to store fat, particularly around the midsection. Even if you're killing it with your diet and exercise, if you're skimping on sleep, your body's stress response could still be setting you up for a metabolic slowdown.

Now, if you're thinking that you function just fine on a few hours of sleep, let's put that thought to rest. While there's a small fraction of the population that can operate well with less sleep, the majority can't cheat the sandman without some metabolic consequence. Those who claim to be immune to sleep's influence might just be too sleep-deprived to notice the deficits.

Adding injury to insult, let's talk about the energy equation. With less sleep, we're more likely to be sedentary—too tired to hit the gym or even take the stairs. The less we move, the fewer calories we burn, mirroring a metabolism that's downshifting into a lower gear. On the flip side, over-compensating with high-sugar or caffeinated products to combat fatigue can result in blood sugar spikes, another metabolic mishap. It's a precarious cycle.

Evidently, getting a full night of quality sleep is more vital than we may have thought, particularly when we're targeting a metabolic reset to lose weight. It's clear that sleep is not just a placeholder between our busy days; it's a crucial player in the symphony of bodily processes that govern our metabolism. So, as we aim for better metabolic health, it's imperative that we make sleep a top priority too.

Lastly, remember that improving sleep quality isn't a luxury; it's a necessity. As we move into our discussion on tips for enhancing sleep, it's vital to understand and respect the intricate dance between sleep and metabolism. Fixing our sleep patterns isn't just about feeling rested—it's about setting our body's metabolic rhythm to its optimal beat.

Tips for Improving Sleep Quality

Sleep, as vital to our metabolism as it is, often becomes the first casualty in our busy lives. It's time to change that because the quality of your sleep can significantly impact your metabolic health. Making small but purposeful adjustments to your sleep habits can set the stage for profound shifts in your overall well-being and weight loss journey.

First things first, let's talk about consistency. Going to bed and waking up at the same time every day can regulate your body's internal clock. It might not sound like much, but this regularity can dramatically enhance sleep quality and, by extension, metabolic efficiency. Think of it as syncing your biological processes for optimal performance.

Next is the ambiance of your bedroom. It should be a sanctuary designed for sleep. Keep it cool, dark, and quiet, and consider if your mattress and pillows are truly serving your comfort. A peaceful environment signals to your brain that it's time to wind down, nudging your metabolism into a restorative state.

Light exposure impacts your sleep more than you might realize. The blue light from screens can interfere with the production of melatonin, your body's sleep hormone. Cutting screen time an hour before bed can make a world of difference in how quickly you fall asleep and the quality of sleep you achieve throughout the night.

Physical activity is a fantastic ally for improving sleep. Regular exercise can deepen your sleep, helping your body's recovery processes, including those involved in metabolism. However, timing is key—aim to finish any vigorous workouts a few hours before bedtime to allow your body to settle back down.

Mind what you eat and drink as the day wanes. A heavy meal right before bed can lead to discomfort and indigestion, both enemies of restful sleep. Similarly, caffeine and alcohol can dramatically disrupt your sleep patterns—even if they seem to make falling asleep easier at first.

If stress is the thief of your rest, explore relaxation techniques like mindfulness, meditation, or deep breathing exercises. These methods can lower your heart rate and prepare your body for sleep, ensuring you're not tossing and turning with racing thoughts.

Consider establishing a **pre-sleep ritual**. This could be anything from reading a book to taking a warm bath. The key is consistency—the ritual becomes a signal to your body that it's time to switch off and drift into restorative slumber.

For some, a pinch of white noise or soothing sounds can be a game-changer. These ambient noises can drown out the jarring sounds of the night or early morning, allowing you to stay enveloped in calm till it's time to wake up refreshed and ready for a new day.

When all else fails, or if you're struggling significantly, don't hesitate to reach out for professional help. Sleep disorders are increasingly common and treatable. Partnering with a healthcare provider can uncover underlying issues that, once addressed, can radically improve your sleep and metabolic health.

Incorporating these sleep optimization tips into your daily routine isn't just about getting more rest—it's about setting up a strong foundation for metabolic success. Improved sleep quality can bolster your energy levels, fortify your resolve for healthy habits, and ultimately aid in resetting your metabolism to lose weight effectively. Sleep isn't just a period of rest; it's when the unseen but crucial work of rejuvenation and balance happens within your body, so prioritize it as much as you would your nutrition and exercise.

The Connection Between Sleep and Appetite

As we delve into the interplay between shut-eye and hunger, it's striking to see how intertwined they truly are, especially when considering metabolism. Sleep—isn't just a period of rest; it's a state that significantly influences our dietary choices and by extension, our metabolic health. Let's break down this intricate relationship.

Starting with appetite regulation—a process that brings hormones into the limelight. Ghrelin, known as the 'hunger hormone', goes up when we lack sleep, making us feel the urge to eat more. On the flip side, leptin, the hormone that tells us we're full, decreases. This hormonal imbalance skews our appetite, and before we know it, we're raiding the kitchen for a midnight snack when what our body truly craves is sleep.

Now, this wouldn't be such a concern if we craved salads and celery sticks, but here's the rub: sleep deprivation increases our penchant for high-calorie, high-carbohydrate foods. It's as if our brain, deprived of the rest it needs to make reasoned choices, falls back on primal urges—urges that equate calories with survival. So, it's not just that we're hungry; we're irrepressibly drawn to the very foods that can derail our metabolism.

Moreover, this cascading effect of a sleep-starved brain doesn't stop at just poor food selection. It's been shown to impair our frontal cortex—where our most considerate decision-making fires—and light up the reward centers of the brain when we see food. In simpler terms, lack of sleep weakens our willpower and intensifies our response to the pleasure we get from eating, especially from sugary or fatty foods.

Let's also not forget the role of circadian rhythms. Our body's natural clock not only dictates our sleep patterns but also our eating habits. Disrupting this rhythm, as poor sleep often does, can result in abnormal eating patterns, which can contribute to weight gain over time, complicating our metabolic well-being.

Think of it this way: Sleep is the guardian of your metabolic balance. When that guardian takes a leave of absence, not only do ghrelin and leptin start pulling the strings in a wayward puppet show of hunger and satiety, but insulin sensitivity can also take a hit. Decreased sleep may lead to higher blood sugar levels and an increased risk for insulin resistance. Remember, insulin is the hormone that plays a key role in our body's ability to use or store the energy from food, thus a crucial player in our metabolic game.

This is where nighttime eating, particularly of carbohydrate-rich foods, complicates the plot. Meals should ideally sync with our body's natural rhythms, but a late-night binge can throw this harmony into chaos, making it harder for insulin to do its job effectively. Thus, eating aligned with a stable sleep pattern helps keep things running more smoothly.

So, if you're looking to reset your metabolism, it's paramount not to ignore the sleep component. After all, a well-rested body is more adept at making smart food choices, portion control, and keeping those pivotal hormones in check. It's not just about the quantity of sleep either; quality matters just as much. Ensuring that your sleep is restorative is a giant leap towards supporting your metabolic goals.

To sum it up, managing sleep is much like tending to the soil in a garden—it's the base from which everything else grows. Neglect it, and you're bound to see weeds—in this case, unfettered appetite and poor food choices—that will hamper the growth of your metabolic health. Nourish it, and you'll reap the benefits of a balanced appetite and a metabolism that runs like a well-oiled machine.

As we close this chapter, consider this: sleep isn't an optional luxury; it's a fundamental aspect of our metabolic system. So, as you endeavor to reset your metabolism, remember that quality zzz's are just as important as the right nutrition and exercise. Embrace sleep as a delightful necessity, and watch how it helps keep your appetite—and metabolism—in harmonious rhythm.

Chapter 10

The Impact of Exercise on Metabolism

Let's dive into the energizing world of physical activity and how it not only reshapes our bodies but supercharges our metabolism too. Now, if you've ever wondered just how going for a run, lifting weights, or even a dynamic yoga session can rev up your metabolic engine, you're in for a real treat. You see, every squat, sprint, and stretch sparks a cascade of metabolic miracles that'll have your body's energy systems firing on all cylinders. We're talking about a serious uptick in calorie burn and a shift towards more efficient energy usage, even when you're lounging post-workout. It's like cranking up your body's inner thermostat—suddenly you're torching calories at a higher rate, all thanks to a bespoke working-out plan. Whether it's heart-pumping cardio or muscle-building strength training, the right mix not only boosts your metabolism but also molds your physique into the powerhouse you deserve. Nudge your gym shoes closer because we're about to embark on a transformative metabolic journey, underlining just how potent exercise is in resetting your body's energy equation.

Different Types of Exercise and Metabolic Effects

Now that we're fired up about umpiring the metabolism game, let's dive into the exercise playbook. Think of your metabolism as a cozy campfire. Just as you can't use big logs alone to get a roaring fire, you can't rely solely on one type of workout to stoke your metabolic flame. Cardio, think brisk walking or cycling, fans the flames, getting that metabolic rate to heat up quickly. It's a calorie-torching sprint at the moment, but the glowing embers don't last as long. On the flip side, strength training, with resistance bands or weights, might not have the same immediate blaze, but it's like adding dense logs that smolder long after the workout ends, meaning your metabolism burns brighter and longer. And don't forget the agility drills—flexibility and balance exercises—because a body that moves well is a body that burns well. So, let's mix it up, shall we? After all, a varied exercise routine doesn't just prevent boredom; it's the secret sauce for a metabolic bonfire that keeps on burning, helping tip the scales in your favor.

Cardiovascular Exercises are the cornerstone of any effective exercise regimen, especially when we talk about resetting your metabolism for weight loss. The heart-pumping, sweat-inducing sessions that you often associate with cardio are essential not only for dropping pounds but also for enhancing your metabolic health. Let's delve into the role cardiovascular workouts play in waking up a sluggish metabolic engine.

Imagine your metabolism is like a fire. To get that fire roaring, you've got to feed it. Cardiovascular workouts are the bellows that pump more air into that metabolic flame, increasing the heat and the intensity of the burn. When you engage in activities like running, swimming, or cycling, you're not just burning calories during the exercise; you're also setting up your body to burn more calories at rest. This process is known as excess post-exercise oxygen consumption, or EPOC for short, and it's your secret weapon in resetting your metabolism.

But it's not about pounding the pavement until you're blue in the face. The key is to find a balance—the right mix of duration, frequency, and intensity that keeps your body guessing and your metabolism churning. For instance, high-intensity interval training (HIIT) is a powerful tool in your cardio toolbox. This type of training alternates between bursts of intense activity and periods of rest or lower intensity. Studies show that HIIT not only torches calories but also improves insulin sensitivity, which is crucial for a healthy metabolism.

On the other hand, don't underestimate the power of steady-state cardio—the longer, moderate-intensity workouts that might include a brisk walk or a leisurely bike ride. While they may not have the explosive calorie-burning effect of HIIT, they're sustainable and can be incredibly beneficial for heart health and endurance building. They're the endurance runs that teach your body to become more efficient at burning fat for fuel, an invaluable skill as one aims to shed excess weight.

Incorporating variety into your cardiovascular exercises is crucial for metabolic adaptation. By varying your workouts, you avoid the dreaded plateau and continue to challenge your body in new ways. One day you might tackle a spin class, and the next take on a dance workout. What's important is that you're moving consistently and with purpose.

Don't forget to tailor your cardio regimen to your current fitness level. If you're starting out, jumping into an intense HIIT session prematurely can lead to injury or burnout. Gradually building up intensity and duration will not only help prevent these setbacks but also ensure sustained progress. Listen to your body—it's the most reliable indicator of how hard you should be pushing yourself.

Cardiovascular exercises also have a profound effect on mental well-being. Exercise releases endorphins, the compound notoriously known for creating a euphoric effect, often referred to as the 'runner's high.' These natural mood lifters can play a vital role in keeping you motivated and committed to your metabolic reset journey. Coupled with the sense of achievement that comes from beating your own personal records, cardio can be as beneficial for your mind as it is for your body.

Let's not forget about the role of cardio in improving sleep quality. Adequate rest is a critical component of metabolic health, and regular cardiovascular activity can help regulate your sleep patterns. Better sleep equates to better recovery, which in turn fuels your ability to consistently engage in effective workouts.

If you've been sedentary for a while, the prospect of incorporating cardiovascular exercises into your routine could seem daunting. It's not about running a marathon on your first day; it's about consistent, gradual improvement. Even a 15-minute walk adds to your metabolic bank. Remember, consistency is key. The regularity of your activity is what will ultimately help reset your metabolism and aid in healthy weight loss.

Wrapping up, cardio is not just a tool for weight loss; it's your partner in reenergizing a sluggish metabolism. Be mindful, though, that cardio is just one aspect of a well-rounded fitness plan. In the following sections, we'll explore the indispensable role of strength training and how to craft an exercise program that balances cardiovascular workouts with muscle-building activities for optimal metabolic health. But for now, understand that lacing up those sneakers and claiming that heartbeat spike is your first step to reinvigorating your metabolic rate and shedding unwanted weight.

Strength Training can feel like an enigma wrapped in spandex. Let's shake that off! If you've been intently nodding along about the role of diet and hormones in metabolic health, prepare for strength training to clinch the deal on resetting your metabolism. If nutrition is the fuel, think of strength training as the engine tune-up your body craves for a ramped-up metabolic rate.

Firstly, understand that muscle is your metabolic ally. Each pound of lean muscle burns more calories at rest than a pound of fat. It's like having a sports car in your garage — it's just naturally fast. When you engage in regular strength training, you're essentially building and maintaining that sports muscle-car, ensuring it burns fuel efficiently, making weight loss less of an uphill battle and more of a scenic cruise.

But let's allay a common fear: bulking up. For most, strength training won't have you bursting through your clothes like the Hulk. Our bodies simply don't spiral into a muscle-building frenzy that easily. Instead, strength training tones and strengthens muscles, which is exactly what your metabolism needs. A toned body is teeming with metabolic potential, the kind that keeps your calorie burn high and your body composition favorable.

Circuit training is a particular gem in the crown of strength training. It involves moving quickly from one exercise to another, targeting different muscle groups with minimal rest in between. The result? You not only build strength but also keep your heart rate up, flirting with the benefits of cardiovascular exercise. It's like sneaking in an extra metabolic kick without your body even realizing it.

Now, diving into specific exercises, compound movements are your best friend. These are exercises like squats, deadlifts, and bench presses that work multiple muscle groups at once. By engaging more muscles, you're demanding more energy, and thus, your metabolism revs up to meet the challenge. Remember, a demanding workout is a respectful nod to your body's capabilities, not a punishment.

Moreover, strength training can be incredibly varied, which means it's adaptable to any fitness level. Start with bodyweight exercises like push-ups and lunges before graduating to resistance bands and then weights. There's no shame in starting light; remember, even the mightiest of oaks sprouted from a humble acorn. The key is progression and consistency, allowing your muscles — and metabolism — to ascend to new heights.

Consider the hormonal symphony that is your body, with strength training being a conductor of sorts. Testosterone and growth hormone, two paramount players in muscle building, are elevated in response to strength training. These are beneficial for both men and women, adding a chisel to muscle and a sizzle to metabolism. Just like any good concert, it's all about harmony and balance.

So, how often should one engage in strength training? Aim for at least 2-3 days per week, ensuring you give your muscles time to recover. They'll be hard at work repairing and growing stronger, which is exactly when your resting metabolic rate decides to strut its stuff. It's within these periods of recovery that your newly developed muscle works its metabolic magic, continuously pressing the burn button on calories, even while you're sprawled out on the couch.

Don't overlook the need for a holistic approach. Yes, strength training is a powerhouse for metabolic health, but it's just one pillar. It thrives alongside a balanced diet, adequate sleep, managed stress, and regular cardiovascular exercises. It's this blend of lifestyle adjustments that sets the stage for a truly effective metabolic reset. You're crafting a symphony, and every element matters in creating that harmonious melody of metabolic health.

In short, strength training isn't merely about getting strong; it's about fostering a foundation for a vibrant metabolism. By incorporating it into your life, you're forging a body more adept at managing weight, with a vitality that extends far beyond the numbers on a scale. It's a tool to transform not only your physique but also your metabolic narrative. So, lift, push, and pull your way to a roaring metabolic engine — one that powers you through life with gusto and verve.

Creating a Balanced Exercise Program

By now, we've grasped how exercise is a formidable ally in revving up our metabolism. But how do we marry different workout styles into a regimen that doesn't just ignite a caloric bonfire but also lays down rich soil for sustainable fitness? It's not just about breaking a sweat; it's about crafting a well-rounded routine that stands the test of time and boredom.

First and foremost, let's deflate a common myth: More isn't always better. Excessive workouts can lead to burnout or, worse, injury. So, when we talk balance, we're referring to a mixture of cardiovascular, strength, and flexibility training, tailored to your unique body and life demands. Think of it as your personal triad of fitness, each pillar supporting and enhancing the other.

When it concerns cardiovascular health, remember moderation and variety. This could be anything from brisk walking to cycling or swimming —

the goal is to get our heart rate up and sustain that increase for a reasonable period. But don't forget the fun factor! Dancing or even participating in team sports can skyrocket your heart rate while keeping a smile plastered on your face.

Moving on to the brawn of the triad: strength training. This is where you challenge your muscles by lifting weights, working with resistance bands, or engaging in bodyweight exercises like push-ups and squats. You don't need to aspire to the physique of bodybuilders, but aiming for two to three sessions a week can do wonders for your muscles and basal metabolic rate.

However, strong muscles need supple joints. Think of flexibility training as the unsung hero that enables the other two to shine. Yoga, Pilates, and targeted stretching workouts shouldn't be afterthoughts but integral components of your balanced program. They can prevent injuries, yes, but they can also improve your exercise performance by increasing your range of motion and decreasing muscle soreness.

Remember, though, your body's response to exercise is as unique as your fingerprint. It's essential to listen to it. Feeling worn down or noticing persistent aches? That might be your cue to take it easy or switch up your activities. Consistency doesn't mean rigidity; it's okay to adapt your exercises to how your body feels on any given day.

Now, let's talk schedule. It's not just about penciling in gym time whenever there's an opening in your calendar. A thoughtful approach means considering the best times to engage in different types of exercises based on your energy levels and lifestyle. Perhaps an early-morning jog to start the day with a bang, weight training in the evening when your muscles are warm, or a weekend yoga session to unwind and rejuvenate — find what works for you.

Moreover, recovery is not a dirty word in the language of a balanced exercise regime. Adequate rest, including quality sleep and active recovery activities like walking or leisurely biking, is compulsory. These periods allow your body to repair, reduce stress hormone levels, and come back stronger.

Let's also squash another pestering notion: You can't out-exercise a bad diet. Integrating proper nutrition and hydration with your workout plan is non-negotiable. They're the building blocks and fuel for your physical endeavors. Skimp on these, and your metabolism could be running on fumes.

Lastly, evaluate and evolve. A balanced program today may need tweaks tomorrow. People change, goals shift, and what once worked, can become stale or less effective. Regularly assessing your routine prevents plateaus and keeps the flame of motivation alive.

In the end, a successful exercise program is one that excites you, challenges you, and, most importantly, is sustainable. It's a beautiful balancing act, one where your metabolism and entire well-being take center stage. A balanced routine is the secret not just for a metabolic reset but for building a lifestyle where fitness seamlessly blends with joy and vitality.

Rest Break

REST BREAK

"There is virtue in work, and there is virtue in rest. Use both and overlook neither." — Alan Cohen

As you'll discover later in the book, rest is essential to any exercise routine. It allows the muscles to repair and grow, adapting to everything you've been training them to do so they can do it even better the next time.

Our brains work a bit like this, too, and you're taking in a ton of information right now. Taking a break to let it seep in while your mind recharges is a valuable use of your time.

By keeping your mind working but taking a step back from the main text for a moment, you're allowing your brain to consolidate all the new information it's learning.

So, how can we turn this rest into an active break to enhance what you're getting from this book? Simple! You can let other people know what you're learning; the upside is that it will help them, too.

By leaving a review of this book on Amazon, you'll show new readers where they can find the guidance they need to master their mindset in order to reach their weight loss goals.

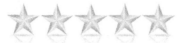

Simply by discussing how this book has helped you and letting other readers know what they'll find inside, you'll show them exactly where to look to find everything they need to leave yo-yo dieting behind forever, and at the same time, your brain will be going over everything you've learned, helping you to embed it in your memory.

Please use the QR code below to leave your review. I appreciate your support. When you're feeling rested and ready to tackle the next chapter, let's move on.

Chapter 11

Understanding and Tackling Weight Loss Plateaus

So you've been following all the advice, eating well, staying active and you've noticed the pounds melting away—until suddenly, it stops. Welcome to the world of weight loss plateaus, a common challenge on the journey to losing weight. But what's really happening with your body and more importantly, how can you overcome this hurdle and get back on track? It's not about working harder; it's about working smarter. In this section, we're delving into the topic of plateaus. We'll explore the reasons behind these stalls—whether it's your body adjusting to a lower calorie intake or small slip ups in your diet consistency. And we'll equip you with practical strategies tailored to revitalize your metabolism, such as adjusting your calorie intake or trying out different exercise routines. By the end of this section, you'll not only understand weight loss plateaus but also have the tools to conquer them and maintain the motivation that initially got you started.

Why Plateaus Happen

Weight loss plateaus can be incredibly frustrating for anyone trying to lose weight—they are where, despite your best efforts, the scale refuses to budge. But what causes these stubborn halts exactly? Understanding the underlying reasons behind plateaus is a crucial step in overcoming them. Initially, when you reduce your calorie intake and increase your exercise regimen, your body reacts by depleting its glycogen stores. These stores serve as quick energy reserves. And shedding water weight since glycogen holds water. This often leads to rapid changes in weight. However, as your body adapts to the reduced calorie intake, it becomes more efficient in utilizing energy, causing your metabolism to slow down and resulting in what we perceive as a plateau in weight loss.

Metabolic adaptation plays a significant role here. Interestingly enough, your own progress contributes to the occurrence of plateaus. The more weight you lose, the less energy your body needs to function. A smaller body burns fewer calories both at rest and during physical activity. It's similar to downsizing from a gas-guzzling SUV to a fuel-efficient compact car; the smaller vehicle simply doesn't need as much fuel to travel the same distance anymore.

Another factor that contributes to plateaus is the loss of lean muscle mass. Often, when people lose weight, they end up losing a combination of fat and muscle tissue. Since muscle burns more calories than fat, losing muscle mass can slow down your metabolic rate.

When you consume fewer calories, your body may use its muscle for energy if it doesn't receive enough fuel from your diet. It's important to avoid relying solely on a specific diet or exercise routine without any variation, as this can contribute to hitting a plateau. By doing the same workout or consuming the same amount of calories every day, your body becomes accustomed to the constant stress. To continue making progress, it is crucial to switch up your routine and keep your body guessing.

It's also essential to consider the impact of hormones. For example, leptin is a hormone that signals feelings of fullness. As you lose fat, leptin levels decrease, which can paradoxically increase appetite and slow down metabolism – an unfavorable combination for weight loss efforts. Other hormones that regulate metabolism and hunger, such as thyroid hormones, insulin, and cortisol, can also influence your weight loss journey.

The quality of your diet plays a significant role as well; it's not just about the quantity but also what you eat. Highly processed foods can disrupt hormone balance and promote insulin resistance. Additionally, diets high in sugar can lead to cravings and compulsive eating habits, making it more challenging to create a calorie deficit.

Psychological factors should not be overlooked either. Stress levels, lack of sleep, and other emotional or environmental factors can affect both your metabolism and willpower.

When you're feeling stressed, your body produces cortisol, which prompts it to conserve energy (i.e., calories). Additionally, if you don't get enough sleep, it can lead to cravings and a decrease in motivation for exercise.

Moreover, we humans are notorious for being bad at estimating how much food we consume and how much exercise we do. Sometimes, what may seem like a weight loss plateau is actually a result of an imbalance between the calories we intake and the calories we burn. Inaccurate tracking of our food intake, underestimating portion sizes, or overestimating the intensity of our workouts can all contribute to this perceived plateau.

Understanding these factors that contribute to weight loss plateaus allows us to develop strategies that directly address them. In the following sections, we will explore ways to overcome these challenges and reignite your weight loss journey. Persistence combined with insight into our body's complex adaptive systems is crucial for overcoming these difficult phases.

It's evident that plateaus are a normal part of the weight loss process; although they can be frustrating at times. However, they should not discourage us as they indicate a need for reassessment and adjustment in our approach. Therefore, it's important not only to anticipate plateaus but also to be prepared for them and know how to adapt when they occur.

Strategies to Break Through a Weight Loss Plateau

Dealing with a weight loss plateau can be quite frustrating during your journey to reset your metabolism. However, don't lose hope! There are effective adjustments you can make to reignite fat burning and get those scales moving again. Let's explore some proven strategies that can help you overcome this obstacle.

Firstly, consider making changes to your diet. You've probably heard about the significance of shaking things up in terms of exercise, right? Well, your nutritional needs aren't much different. Occasionally modifying your intake of macronutrients or micronutrients can surprise your body and give metabolism a boost. If you've been cutting back on carbohydrates lately, it might be time to reintroduce them sensibly into your diet.

Next, let's discuss the importance of strength training. If you've primarily focused on cardio exercises, incorporating or increasing strength training can make a significant difference. Muscles act as metabolic engines that burn calories even at rest. Building more muscle is like upgrading your body's engine to burn more fuel.

Intermittent fasting is another approach that has the potential to revitalize weight loss efforts. By alternating between periods of eating and fasting, you may enhance insulin sensitivity and increase levels of human growth hormone—both essential factors for losing fat.

It's important to explore different fasting schedules to find one that suits your lifestyle and how your body responds. Also, don't underestimate the impact of sleep on your weight loss journey. Poor sleep can disrupt your appetite hormones, leading to increased hunger and cravings. By focusing on good sleep habits, such as having a regular bedtime and reducing screen time before bed, you can regulate these hormones and support your weight loss efforts.

Another approach is to reassess your hydration habits. Water is like the lubricant for your body's machinery, keeping everything running smoothly. Additionally, drinking enough water can boost your metabolism and help you feel fuller before meals, potentially reducing overall calorie intake.

Managing stress is also crucial. Chronic stress can lead to elevated levels of cortisol. A hormone linked to weight gain, particularly around the midsection. Incorporating relaxation techniques such as deep breathing exercises, yoga, or meditation into your routine can help manage stress levels effectively.

It's also possible that you may be consuming more calories than you realize; this is a common issue and not indicative of failure. Consider keeping a food diary or using an app to track your food.

Being mindful of your portion sizes and accurately tracking your food intake can help you uncover hidden calories that might be contributing to the plateau you're experiencing. It's important to consider that a plateau could indicate a need to adjust your expectations. Even if the number on the scale isn't changing, changes in body composition could mean that you're still making progress by losing inches. Look beyond the scale and consider taking measurements or focusing on how your clothes fit as alternative ways to assess your progress.

If you've tried various strategies without success, it might be worth seeking guidance from a professional such as a dietitian or personal trainer. They can provide personalized advice based on a detailed assessment of your diet, exercise routine, and lifestyle habits, helping you overcome plateaus.

Remember, hitting a plateau doesn't mean you've reached the end of your journey; instead, it presents an opportunity for growth and change. By implementing these strategies, you're not solely focused on losing another pound but also fostering healthier metabolic habits. A plateau can become a turning point that propels you towards long-lasting transformation and optimal well-being.

Maintaining Motivation

Maintaining motivation is often one of the most challenging aspects throughout this transformative journey—especially when progress seems stagnant due to plateaus on the scale. It's crucial to understand that sustained weight loss and resetting metabolism are about strategy and winning the psychological battle to keep moving forward.

So, how do you keep that flame burning? First and foremost, it's important to understand that encountering plateaus is a normal and expected part of the process. Mentally preparing yourself for these temporary setbacks can go a long way. They are simply your body's way of adjusting to change, so it's crucial to remind yourself that you haven't failed; your body is just adapting.

Another game-changing strategy is focusing on non scale victories. While the numbers on the scale may fluctuate and sometimes deceive, there are other measures of success that are more reliable indicators of progress. Consider how your clothes fit, the increase in energy levels, or improvements in sleep quality. These factors can provide a more accurate reflection of the positive changes you're making.

Never underestimate the power of remembering "why" you started this journey. On those challenging days when doubt creeps in, reconnect with the reasons that initially motivated you. It could be for better health to enjoy quality time with loved ones or striving for a stronger self image. The deeper your underlying motivation, the more difficult it becomes to let go.

Building a support system is an invaluable asset along this journey. Surrounding yourself with people who genuinely support and believe in you can make all the difference when facing tough times. Whether it's friends, family members, or becoming part of an online community, having cheerleaders in your corner can reignite your determination to overcome challenges.

Lastly, visualization can be an incredibly powerful tool in achieving your goals.

Imagine envisioning yourself in the future, enjoying the fruits of your hard work. This visualization can give you an instant boost of motivation whenever you need it. Consider creating a vision board or practicing meditation to help keep your goals at the forefront of your mind.

Flexibility plays a crucial role in maintaining high levels of motivation. When you encounter a plateau, it's beneficial to shake things up a bit. Try incorporating new workout routines or making small adjustments to your diet; these changes can reignite your body's response to your efforts. Don't be afraid to deviate from your original plan; instead, focus on finding what works best for you in the long run.

Embrace curiosity as a friend during plateaus. Treat them as opportunities to dive deeper into understanding how your body responds to different dietary and lifestyle adjustments. Keeping a journal can be incredibly helpful in tracking and documenting these discoveries, serving as a written testament of your personal journey that you can reflect upon.

Lastly, make sure to celebrate every step forward, no matter how small it may seem. Rewarding yourself for sticking with it, even during challenging times, reinforces the positive habits and behaviors you're developing along the way. Choose rewards that align with your goals—a massage after achieving milestones or acquiring new fitness accessories that enhance your workouts are great examples.

When all these aspects come together harmoniously, they pave the way for an enduring metabolic reset journey.

Even if the numbers on the scale don't change, you're still making progress in transforming your physical appearance, attitude towards health, and perseverance. This journey is about building a strong mindset just as much as it is about losing weight and improving your metabolism. So when you face a plateau, don't allow it to discourage you—use it as motivation to become an even stronger and more determined version of yourself.

Chapter 12

Metabolism-Boosting Supplements

As we move from understanding the crucial role of lifestyle changes in rejuvenating our metabolism, Chapter 12 ventures into the realm of metabolism-boosting supplements. You've got the diet and exercise down, but maybe you're searching for that extra edge. This section isn't a panacea, but a realistic look at supplements that can aid you in your quest to lose weight. We're going to sift through the noise and provide insights into what's safe, what's effective, and how adaptogens might just be the unsung heroes in your metabolic symphony. It's not about popping pills willy-nilly; it's about carefully selecting supplements that work harmoniously with your body's natural processes. Think of this chapter as a guide on when to give your body that supplemental nudge, helping you stride past common hurdles with scientifically backed support. Just remember, supplements are a companion to—not a replacement for—solid nutritional and exercise practices.

Safe and Effective Supplements

After navigating the vast landscape of metabolic enhancers, it's critical to hone in on what truly matters: safe and effective supplements. It's a wild world in the supplement market; a reasonable approach is imperative. Let's cut through the hype and zero in on those that are backed by credible science and have stood the test of practical application.

First up are omega-3 fatty acids. These powerful compounds do more than just support heart health; they may also aid in boosting metabolic rates. Omega-3s, found in fish oil or algal oil for the vegetarians in the room, are fats that your body can't make on its own. Integrating these into your diet can help reduce inflammation, which is often a hidden handbrake to an efficient metabolism.

Protein powders, while not a magic potion, serve as a convenient tool in your metabolic tool belt. They can help repair and build muscle tissue, particularly after a workout, nudging your metabolism to work a bit harder. When it comes to protein supplements, whey, casein, and plant-based options each have their merits. Just ensure you're not hitching a ride on the high-sugar train that some protein products are conducting.

Don't overlook the importance of vitamin D. Studies suggest a correlation between higher levels of vitamin D and metabolic health. Given that the sun remains the most prolific supplier of this nutrient and our indoor lifestyles limit exposure, a supplement can be a key ally. Vitamin D functions like a hormone in the body, playing roles from mood regulation to calcium absorption.

Then there's green tea extract, a source of caffeine and catechins. This dynamic duo fires up the furnace of your metabolism, potentially leading to increased fat burn, especially around the midsection. The most active catechin, EGCG, has received nods for its thermogenic properties. Yet, remember, moderation is key. High doses of green tea extract can be hard on the liver.

On the subject of thermogenesis, capsaicin—the compound that gives peppers their heat—could also add some spark to your metabolic flame. Available in supplement form, capsaicin is said to boost the number of calories burned after consumption. Be mindful, though, of the spicy journey it takes your digestive system on, and balance it with your tolerance.

Magnesium is the unsung hero of mineral supplements, playing a supporting role in over 300 enzyme reactions in the human body. It has its fingers in many pies, from energy production to muscle function. Considering that many individuals fall short of the recommended magnesium intake, a supplement here might not just aid in metabolic health but overall well-being too.

The B vitamins, often grouped together in complexes, are another cast of characters important for a functioning metabolism. Collectively, they assist in the conversion of food into energy. Look for B-complex supplements that contain all eight B vitamins—at reasonable doses, no less—for a more harmonious metabolic symphony.

Fiber supplements, such as psyllium husk or glucomannan, can support metabolic health indirectly by promoting satiety and digestive regularity. They may not rev up your metabolism per se, but by helping you feel fuller for longer, you're less likely to overeat, thus supporting your overall strategy.

Finally, remember that supplements are not a standalone solution. They work best when part of a broader metabolic reset that includes nourishing foods, ample sleep, meaningful movement, and stress management. Always consult with a healthcare professional before starting any new supplement regime, particularly if you're pregnant, nursing, or have existing health conditions.

In conclusion, while these supplements could construct a more efficient metabolism, integrating them should be a move made with informed caution. They're channels to potentially elevate your metabolic baseline, not crutches to lean on for weight loss. Strive for a balance, pay close attention to your body's responses, and build a lifestyle that supports your metabolism through diet, exercise, and mindfulness practices.

The Role of Adaptogens

As we delve into the milieu of metabolism-boosting supplements, an intriguing group emerges that has sparked keen interest in both traditional and modern health circles: adaptogens. These natural substances play a significant role in the narrative of metabolic health, and for good reason. Let's explore their nuanced performance.

Adaptogens, by their nature, are a select class of herbs and mushrooms that support the body's natural ability to handle stress. Stress isn't just about the psychological whirlwinds we face; it's also about the physiological tempests that can decelerate our metabolic functions. These botanicals assist in normalizing our body's processes and can gently nudge our metabolism onto a more favorable path.

Let's get specific. There's a two-way street of influence when we talk about metabolism and adaptogens. These plants help in modulating the adrenal system, which can directly affect our metabolic rate. You see, when the body is inundated with stress, cortisol levels spike, and this can disrupt the metabolic balance. Adaptogens work to temper cortisol, potentially easing the body back into metabolic harmony.

Take, for instance, Ashwagandha. It's a heavyweight in the world of adaptogens and has been studied for its potential to enhance stamina and reduce stress. Less stress equals lower cortisol, and potentially, a more active metabolism. Ginseng is another player with a reputation for boosting energy and aiding in the fight against fatigue.

Now, you might be thinking, can I just load up on adaptogens and watch the magic happen? It's crucial to understand they're not overnight miracles. Adaptogens work subtly, and their strengths lie in their ability to provide cumulative benefits. It's about the long game, investing in a botanical alliance that supports resilience against stress over time.

Moreover, adaptogens don't hoard the spotlight; they're part of an ensemble cast. Think about how they can harmonize with a diverse nutrient profile from your diet or other supplements tailored to metabolic health. For example, pairing adaptogens with micronutrients that support thyroid function can amplify your metabolic strategy.

But let's not wander through the adaptogens garden without precautions. Although natural, these herbs are potent and need to be dosed and taken judiciously. It's a conversation to have with a healthcare provider, ensuring they harmonize with your unique bodily orchestra and don't drown out any other instrument playing its part for your metabolic health.

Considering the consumer landscape, it's clear the market is blooming with adaptogenic offerings. But not all products are created equal. Quality and sourcing matter, because the efficacy of adaptogens can be diluted by poor extraction methods or unsavory additives. Look for products with transparent sourcing and standardized extract labels to really get what you're bargaining for.

The beautiful dance of adaptogens with your metabolism also extends beyond capsules and powders. These adaptogens can be found woven into different teas or culinary dishes, offering a compelling way to diversify your metabolic toolkit and pleasure your palate in the process.

In closing, as with any supplement aimed at boosting metabolism, adaptogens should be integrated as part of a holistic approach. It's about creating a symphony where each instrument—diet, exercise, sleep, and stress management—plays a vital role. Adaptogens can be an exquisite addition to this metabolic concert, but they perform best when the entire orchestra is in tune.

When to Use Supplements

So, you've been on this metabolic journey, tracing how everything from your hormones to your gut health weaves the complex tapestry of your metabolic health. You're now wondering, "Where do supplements fit into this?" Well, let's clear the air. Supplements are not a magic solution, but they can be a valuable tool when used appropriately. Let's talk about when it might be time to consider adding them to your metabolic reset plan.

First off, if you're like many people, you might hit a plateau during your weight loss journey. This can be mentally challenging and baffling, especially when you feel like you're doing everything right. Supplements, particularly those proven to aid in metabolism, could be just the strategic push your body needs to get over that hump. But remember, they work best in conjunction with a healthy diet and regular exercise. There are no shortcuts around those cornerstones!

Another reason to consider supplementation? Nutritional deficiencies. Try as you might; ensuring a perfectly balanced diet every day is tough. There are just times when life gets in the way. Maybe you had to skip lunch for that marathon meeting, or perhaps fresh produce isn't as readily available. If your diet can't provide the essential nutrients necessary for a thriving metabolism, a well-chosen supplement may be in order.

Now, let's talk specifics. Certain supplements have been shown to support metabolic function directly. However, remember, their effectiveness can be influenced by your individual nutritional needs and health conditions. Always talk to a healthcare provider before starting a new supplement.

If you're not sure whether you need supplements, consider getting a comprehensive checkup. Blood tests can reveal a lot about your nutritional status and pinpoint any glaring gaps in your diet. You see, your body speaks to you through numbers and markers, sometimes whispering, sometimes shouting that it's short on certain nutrients. Listening to those signals is key.

Stress. It doesn't do your metabolism any favors. When life's pressures are relentless, something called adaptogens—think of them as your body's stress buffers—help manage the impact on your metabolic health. Incorporating adaptogens through supplements might provide the necessary balance for those too-frequent stressful days.

But be cautious; don't use supplements as a crutch to justify an otherwise unhealthy lifestyle. No supplement can outrun a bad diet or erase the consequences of insufficient sleep and exercise. They are not a license to indulge but a helping hand to guide you towards better overall health.

For the fitness enthusiasts striving for peak performance or individuals engaged in heavy physical labor, supplements can bolster your energy levels and aid muscle recovery. Muscles that are well-nourished and cared for will, in turn, contribute to a higher metabolic rate and more efficient calorie burn.

Let's also consider age. Despite our best efforts, as we get older, our bodies don't always absorb nutrients as well or perform as efficiently. Supplements might mitigate this natural decline, supporting a metabolism that's facing the hurdles of aging.

Ultimately, supplements are about filling in the gaps and giving your body what it needs to triumph in the metabolic marathon. They can be a great addition when your dietary intake falls short or when you need an extra nudge towards your goals. But like all powerful tools, they must be used wisely and with knowledge of their time and place. Ensure any metabolic supplement you introduce to your regime serves a purpose and complements the bigger picture of your health.

So, as you progress on your journey to reset your metabolism, remember that supplements are a supplement—not a replacement—to the foundational elements of proper nutrition, sufficient sleep, regular physical activity, and stress management. With that mindset, they can be a valuable ally in reaching your weight loss and health objectives.

Chapter 13

Meal Planning for Metabolic Health

Now that we've primed our bodies with the tools and knowledge of a metabolic reset, let's dive into what's cooking in Chapter 13: Meal Planning for Metabolic Health. We're going to throw out the notion that healthy eating is bland and overly complicated. It's time to fuel that internal furnace with meal plans that pack a punch for your metabolism without chaining you to the kitchen counter. Think of it as crafting a daily menu that makes your cells dance and your energy levels surge. Remember, we're not just counting calories; we're making calories count. We'll lay out the essentials of a metabolically minded menu teeming with variety, flavor, and nutritional balance. We'll look at how to harmonize with your body's clock without feeling deprived. Gone are the days of scouring the web for "metabolic recipes" only to find yourself lost in a rabbit hole of contradictory advice. We'll provide practical, simple-to-prepare dishes that work with your schedule, not against it. So, let's stock our pantries and crank up the heat—it's time to plan meals that not only taste delicious but rocket your metabolic health to new heights!

Basics of Metabolically Minded Meal Planning

So, we've talked about the nuts and bolts of metabolism, and you've got the basic idea that what you eat—and how you eat it—can crank up that metabolic fire. Now, let's get down to brass tacks and talk about how to plan your meals to keep the fire burning and stoke it like a pro.

First things first, let's get real about carbs. You can't avoid them, and you shouldn't want to—they're your body's preferred source of energy. But let's be smart about it. Go for carbs that release energy nice and slow, things like whole grains, legumes, and veggies. The aim is to avoid blood sugar spikes that can mess with your hormones and keep your metabolism guessing.

Now, fats have gotten a bad rap, but they're essential for good metabolism. The key is choosing the right ones and nixing the wrong. Say yes to sources like avocados, nuts, seeds, and fatty fish. These guys are packed with omega-rich goodness that supports a healthy metabolism, and they keep you feeling full longer, so you're less likely to snack on junk.

Let's not forget protein. It's the building block of muscle, and muscle is like metabolic currency. The more you have, the richer you are in burning calories. So, ensure you've got a good source of protein with every meal. You don't have to go overboard—just a consistent supply throughout the day to maintain muscle mass and keep that metabolic rate up.

Remember, no nutrient lives in isolation. They're a team, working together to keep you running like a well-oiled machine. So, when you're planning your meals, think diversity. A rainbow of veggies, various protein sources (meat, fish, tofu, beans), and whole grains like quinoa and farro will get you all those vital nutrients that keep the engine running smoothly.

Timing is everything, right? The same goes for eating. Regular meal times can be just as crucial as what's on your plate. By eating at consistent times, you're giving your metabolism regular cues, letting it know that it's got the energy to work with, and there's no need to hit the panic button and start conserving calories.

Hydration can't be overstated. It's not just about quenching thirst; water is essential for metabolic processes. Sipping on water throughout the day can help keep your metabolic engine from overheating and seizing up. It's like keeping your car topped off with coolant—it just runs better.

Portion control isn't about restriction; it's about understanding your body's needs. Eating more than necessary can lead to weight gain, sure, but under-eating can slow your metabolism as your body tries to conserve energy. Find that Goldilocks zone where you're eating just right for your activity level.

Let's talk about meal composition. Each meal should have that perfect symphony of macros and micros I mentioned. But also, the texture and flavor play a role in satiety—that feeling of being full and satisfied. You can't just eat cardboard-tasting food and expect to stick with it. Spice things up, literally, and enjoy the flavors of what you eat. It'll help you stick to the plan if you actually like what you're consuming!

And hey, I know life is hectic. Meal prep can be a lifesaver. Dedicating a few hours to prepare your meals for the week can make sure you're eating what you should be when you should be. You're less likely to grab a calorie-dense, nutrient-poor option if you've got a home-cooked meal waiting for you.

Last up, flexibility is your friend. You're human. There will be days when you sway from the path. But here's the thing: One off-track meal or day is not going to undo all your hard work. So don't sweat it. Get right back on it with the next meal or day. Structured flexibility can make this metabolic-minded meal planning a sustainable part of your life.

Sample Meal Plans

Navigating the terrain of metabolic health doesn't have to be a trek through the unknown. With a solid meal plan as your map, you're well on your way to resetting your metabolism and embarking on a more energized lifestyle. Here, we'll lay out some sample meal plans that'll not only nourish your body but also cater to your taste buds. After all, a diet that's both delicious and nutritionally dense is more like a joy ride than a chore.

Think of your first meal of the day as the initial burst of fuel that ignites your metabolic engine. A breakfast that's rich in proteins and fats can provide sustained energy without spiking blood sugar levels. Imagine starting your day with a spinach and feta omelet paired with a side of avocado. Not only will this keep you full, but it also sets the tone for a day of smart eating choices.

Lunch is the perfect time to incorporate lean proteins and a rainbow of vegetables to keep your metabolism humming. A quinoa salad tossed with grilled chicken, cherry tomatoes, cucumbers, red onions, and a lemon-tahini dressing packs a flavorful punch while delivering the necessary nutrients to support your metabolic functions.

When mid-afternoon hunger strikes, reach for snacks that combine fiber with protein. Greek yogurt with a handful of almonds and a sprinkle of chia seeds can curb those hunger pangs without derailing your metabolism from its peak performance.

Dinners in our meal plan are anything but dull. They're designed to satisfy you while optimizing your metabolic health. Picture a plate of seared salmon, its omega-3 fatty acids playing a vital role in hormone balance, alongside a heap of roasted Brussels sprouts drizzled with olive oil for that added antioxidant boost. This kind of meal not only tantalizes the taste buds but also supports your body's natural repair processes overnight.

Now, no one's saying you can't enjoy a treat here and there. The key is to choose desserts that are as beneficial as they are indulgent. A small bowl of mixed berries with a dollop of whipped coconut cream offers a sweet ending without a blood sugar spike.

Hydration also plays a crucial role in metabolic health, so don't forget to drink plenty of water throughout the day. Infuse it with slices of citrus or cucumber for an extra flavor dimension and refreshing twist.

Each meal and snack in this plan has been chosen to ensure a steady supply of energy and nutrients. By focusing on whole, unprocessed foods, you're providing your body with the high-quality fuel it needs to perform at its best—like tuning a high-performance vehicle with the finest grade of gasoline.

And this is just to get your gears turning; the possibilities for crafting satisfying, metabolic-friendly meals are endless. Once you familiarize yourself with the concepts from earlier chapters—like the importance of balancing macronutrients and the role of gut health—these sample plans can be a launchpad for your culinary creativity.

Remember, you're not just eating to fill a gap—you're cultivating a relationship with food that energizes and empowers your body. This is where metabolic magic happens—where smart dietary choices transform into noticeable boosts in energy and weight management success. Let these meal plan samples be your stepping stones to a more vibrant, healthier you.

With flavors to look forward to and nutrients that are in it for the long haul, you're setting the stage for a metabolic reboot that's as sustainable as it is scrumptious. These sample meal plans combine solid science with a love for good food, creating a harmony between health and pleasure. That's the heart of a sustainable lifestyle choice—one that celebrates every meal as an opportunity for nourishment and joy.

Chapter 14

Tracking Your Progress

So, you've revamped your diet, tuned into your body's needs, and established an exercise rhythm that feels just right. Now, let's focus on gauging the fruits of your steadfast dedication with 'Tracking Your Progress.' Imagine having a compass that ensures you're not just going in circles but actually forging ahead—that's what tracking does for your weight loss journey. It's not simply about the numbers on the scale; it's about understanding the nuances of your body's responses and adapting accordingly. We'll dive into the significance of regular monitoring, from jotting down your meals to noting the fluctuations in your energy levels. You'll discover tools that seamlessly align with this pursuit—fitness apps that feel like a personal coach in your pocket and wearables that whisper insights about your health with every step. These aren't just gadgets and journals; they're your allies in the quest to strike metabolic harmony. So, let's not leave our progress to guesswork; let's measure, refine, and celebrate every victory and insight on this transformative escapade.

The Importance of Monitoring

As we've navigated the nuances of resetting your metabolism, weight loss surfaces as both an art and a science. An essential brushstroke in this masterpiece is monitoring your progress. You see, this isn't simply about stepping on a scale—it's about forming a narrative that captures your metabolic rewrite.

Think about why skyscrapers don't sway in the breeze or why bridges don't collapse under weight—it's the meticulous attention to detail during construction. Similarly, monitoring your journey ensures the foundation of your metabolic reset is solid. Here's a revelation: the scale, while a tool, isn't the end-all. It's only a small part of your health portfolio.

By keeping tabs on various aspects of your health, you get invaluable feedback. Are you getting stronger? Is your energy level soaring? Do you see an improvement in your sleep quality? Monitoring isn't just about numbers; it's about quality of life.

Tracking food intake isn't about restriction, but about understanding which foods serve your metabolic goals. These insights help you make more informed choices, transforming diets from a guessing game to a strategic plan that fuels your body efficiently.

What about exercise? Recording workouts helps you level up gradually, preventing plateaus from becoming permanent residents in your fitness journey. By assessing the type, duration, and intensity of your workouts, you can adjust your routine to maximize metabolic benefits.

Let's not ignore the silent player: stress. Its covert operations can derail your metabolic train without a trace. Keeping a log of your stress levels, and understanding how they correlate with dietary choices and weight fluctuations, can lead to better mental and physical health management strategies.

Blood tests take on a whole new meaning when you're in tune with your metabolic health. Instead of a bi-annual surprise, it's a graded paper showcasing the results of your hard work—or indicating where you need to double down on your efforts.

Photos and measurements also tell a story more profound than a number on the scale. As your body composition evolves, the mirror becomes a friend, reflecting muscles and curves where there used to be none—tangible proof that you're sculpting a new you.

Lastly, let's address the emotional and psychological measurements—arguably the most significant ones. How's your mood on most days? Are you more resilient? By observing these subjective aspects, we understand systemic metabolic health and how it infiltrates every facet of our being.

In conclusion, monitoring is the compass that guides you through the jungle of misinformation and keeps you on the path to success. It goes beyond vanity and numbers; it's a comprehensive approach that integrates the physical, mental, and emotional strides you're making. It's not just about losing weight—it's about gaining a whole new perspective on life.

Tools and Techniques for Tracking

Mastery over your metabolic reset journey requires a diligent awareness of your progression. Let's get straight into how you can effectively track your advances with tools and techniques designed to offer clarity and insight into your transformation. The goal is simple: arm yourself with the best instruments to capture the nuances of your progress.

Firstly, consider the classic—journaling. There's an undeniable power in the pen that takes your journey from intangible to concrete. Regularly jotting down your dietary intake, exercise routines, energy levels, and emotional well-being provides a canvas upon which your metabolic story unfolds. Remember, the devil's in the details, so the more meticulous your records, the clearer the patterns of what works for you will emerge.

The scale can be a double-edged sword, but when used thoughtfully, it's a valuable ally. Weighing yourself shouldn't be a daily obsession, but a weekly check-in can be revealing. Be aware, however, that weight can be deceptive, masking the subtleties of fat loss and muscle gain, which is why the tape measure is another vital companion. Circumference measurements of your waist, hips, and other body parts can indicate shifts in body composition often missed by the scale alone.

Let's not forget technology, which has revolutionized self-monitoring. Fitness apps and wearables track and crunch data like steps taken, calories burned, sleep quality, and much more. By converting your daily activities into actionable insights, they illuminate the path and sway you towards smarter, more informed decisions.

Then there is perhaps one of the most telling methods of gauging progress: how your clothes fit. It's a tangible metric that provides immediate feedback—no charts or numbers needed. If your once-snug jeans are now slipping off your hips or your favorite belt needs an extra notch, you're likely on the right track.

Photos are another potent tracking device. A picture captures more than a moment; it captures the physical transformation unfolding over time. Take consistent progress photos in the same attire and settings to visualize the changes that numbers alone can't describe.

Body fat percentage measurements also offer a glimpse into your metabolic shift. Tools like skin calipers or more advanced body composition scales can provide deeper insights into your fat-to-muscle ratio, highlighting not just weight loss but also the healthy development of muscle mass that keeps your metabolism humming.

While self-monitoring is vital, professional assessments have their place too. Periodic check-ups with your health professional using blood tests, among other evaluations, can confirm the internal metabolic changes that correspond with your dietary and lifestyle adjustments.

But remember, the most critical tool at your disposal is your body's feedback. Listen intently to what it's telling you. Are you energized? Sleep well? Does your body feel lighter and more agile? These qualitative measures are prime indicators that your metabolic reset is doing its magic.

Utilize a combination of these tools to tailor a tracking regime that's as unique as your journey. No single method is definitive, but together, they provide a mosaic of metrics, painting a detailed picture of your metabolic success. With persistence and patience, the data you amass will guide your path toward not just a lighter frame, but a vibrant, rejuvenated life.

So, take the reigns and measure what matters—progress, in its many forms, awaits your acknowledgment. And as we gaze into the next chapter, we'll explore how these tools and techniques can further dovetail with fitness apps and wearables to enrich our understanding of our journey towards a heightened metabolic function.

Fitness Apps and Wearables

In the modern quest for peak metabolic performance and weight loss, technology has become an indispensable ally. The fusion of fitness apps and wearable devices represents a revolution in the way we approach our health goals. If you're ready to reset your metabolism and shed pounds, weaving these digital tools into the fabric of your lifestyle can be your game-changer.

Think of fitness apps as your pocket-sized personal trainers. They offer a plethora of features, from tracking caloric intake to providing customized workout recommendations. More than that, they serve up a motivational feast—reminding you to stand up, move around, log your meals, and stay hydrated. It's about making data work for you, with every bite and every step calculated towards your metabolic reset.

Wearables go a step further. They cling to your wrist, sit tight on your waist, or even snug up in your running shoes, diligently monitoring your every move. The real magic happens when these devices translate physical activity into readable metrics—your heartbeat, steps taken, and calories burned. They show you the raw evidence of what happens to your body when you're on the move versus when you're not. Remember, the goal here isn't just an activity; it's an informed activity that aligns with metabolic enhancement.

What's crucial about these apps and devices is not the sheer volume of data they provide but the insights into your personal habits. They break down the barriers of self-reporting error and delusion by giving you undeniable metrics—how much you actually move versus how much you think you move. Over time, this eradicates guesswork and helps paint a more accurate picture of your lifestyle and its impact on your metabolism.

Syncing your digital tools with specific goals can be thrilling, too. Are you looking to increase your muscle mass and thereby contribute to a higher basal metabolic rate? Your wearables can monitor your strength training progress, ensuring you're hitting the right intensities and rest periods. Curious if you're truly doing enough cardio to enhance your metabolic flexibility? The app is there to keep track and keep you on a path that complements your dietary changes.

The social facets these apps foster should not be underestimated. Many can connect you with communities who share similar goals, challenges, and victories. This sense of camaraderie, which transcends the isolation of personal fitness journeys, can be a source of tremendous support. Knowing others are celebrating your milestones and pushing through similar struggles reinforces commitment and accountability.

When used thoughtfully, fitness apps and wearables provide actionable feedback. They allow for a level of fine-tuning to your exercise routine that was once only available in professional athletic facilities. Finding out that your heart rate doesn't quite reach your target zone during a supposed high-intensity workout could be the catalyst for adjusting and optimizing your regimen for better fat burn and metabolic outcomes.

It's not just about higher, faster, stronger, though. Recovery is as important as the activity itself, especially when it comes to metabolic health. Wearables now come armed with features tracking your sleep patterns, stress levels, and even suggesting recovery times. This sort of holistic approach is key in ensuring that your metabolism doesn't just spike and dip but evolves into a finely tuned engine burning fuel efficiently.

However, amidst this digital enthusiasm, we must remember that apps and wearables offer support, not solutions. They're a means to an end. The tech should empower, not overwhelm. It's easy to get lost in numbers and graphs, but your focus should be on how these tools can foster better habits and, ultimately, a better understanding of your metabolic health.

A metabolism reset isn't a passive process—it's active, it's dynamic, and it's uniquely tailored to you. Incorporating fitness apps and wearables into this journey places a compass in your hand, guiding you towards informed decisions and meaningful progress in your health voyage. So, embrace these tech companions as you turn every stride, every rep, and every meal into a step towards a rebooted metabolism and a rejuvenated you.

Chapter 15

Building Sustainable Habits

As we shift gears from tracking progress to establishing the cornerstone of long-term success, it's critical to delve into the science of habit formation and figure out how to turn temporary changes into lifelong routines. It's all about getting those neural pathways in your brain to recognize your healthy choices as default behaviors. These are actions that, once ingrained, don't require a second thought, like reaching for water instead of soda or gearing up for a brisk walk without the inner groan. With the guidance laid out in previous chapters, you've got the foundation—now, let's reinforce those structures. Whether you're someone who thrives on the slow-steady-wins-the-race approach or you prefer quantum leaps, this chapter is where you'll learn to cement those healthy decisions day after day until they're as natural to you as breathing. After all, consistency is your ally, not just in metabolic reset but also in carving out a life brimming with vitality and vigor.

The Psychology of Habit Formation

As we embark on the journey of reshaping our daily routines to support a healthy metabolism, it's essential to understand the psychology that underpins habit formation. Habits, those automatic behaviors we perform almost without thinking, are the bedrock of daily life. They are the brain's way of saving energy by relegating routine tasks to autopilot, freeing up mental resources for more complex challenges. Yet, while habits can be incredibly beneficial, they can also be stubborn to change—especially when they're linked to deeply ingrained patterns of eating or activity.

What is intriguing about habits is that they are underpinned by a simple yet profound loop consisting of a cue, a routine, and a reward. This loop is at the core of why habits, once established, can become so automatic. When it comes to metabolic health, the power lies in hacking this loop to foster habits that align with our goals for weight management and energy level enhancement. Imagine this: every time you feel a late-night craving (the cue), instead of reaching for a sugary snack, you opt for a glass of water or a healthier alternative (the routine), and in doing so, you experience a sense of self-fulfillment (the reward). What begins as a conscious choice can, with repetition, evolve into a natural part of your daily rhythm.

To make this transformation successful, it's vital to focus initially on the cues that trigger our less desired habits. This means setting up your environment to reduce temptations and crafting new cues that signal the start of positive routines. For example, laying out your workout clothes the night before can become a visual cue to prioritize exercise in the morning. Similarly, preparing your workspace with healthy snacks can steer you clear of the vending machine when the mid-afternoon slump hits. Creating these visual or sensory triggers can be the nudge we need to flip the switch on healthier behavior patterns.

Then comes the challenge of consistency. Every time you repeat a healthy routine in response to a cue and savor the reward that follows, you're one step closer to cementing a habit. It's not always going to be a smooth path—the initial rewards of lifestyle change, such as feeling more energetic or noticing a dip in the scale, can plateau, and that's when the risk of backsliding looms largest. Combatting this requires doubling down on mindful awareness of the rewards that extend beyond the immediate and tangible. The long-term payoffs, like improved overall health, a sense of achievement, and a more robust metabolic state, are rewards potent enough to keep the habit loop spinning.

Finally, let's consider the social and emotional components of habit formation. Emotional states can serve as powerful cues, and our social environments can profoundly influence our routines. By aligning your surroundings with your goals and seeking support from friends or family members who cheer for your progress, you're setting the stage for positive reinforcement that makes the new habits stick. It's about crafting a personal ecosystem where healthy choices are the easiest to make and where each step towards metabolic health is celebrated as a victory in its own right.

Tips for Establishing and Maintaining Healthy Habits

Now that we've delved into the intricacies of metabolism and how various factors can either support or inhibit its proper function, let's pivot to the practical actions that you can take day-to-day. As we know, starting with new habits is one thing, but the real magic lies in their maintenance. So, how do we translate bursts of motivation into long-standing patterns of behavior? Let's talk strategy.

First and foremost, start small. It might seem counterintuitive when you're chomping at the bit to make big changes, but bite-sized habits are more digestible and sustainable. For instance, if you want to increase your activity level, you might begin with a daily 10-minute walk rather than attempting a full-blown hour at the gym. These manageable commitments can quickly morph into cornerstones of your daily routine without overwhelming you.

Consistency is key, but so is flexibility. That might sound like a contradiction, but here's the thing - life isn't predictable, and your habits shouldn't be so rigid that they break under the slightest pressure. If you miss a workout or indulge in a treat, don't throw in the towel. Adapt and move forward. Tomorrow is a fresh opportunity to reaffirm your commitment to your goals.

Speaking of goals, let's make them SMART: Specific, Measurable, Achievable, Relevant, and Time-bound. Aiming to 'lose weight' is too vague. Instead, aim to 'lose 5 pounds in one month by incorporating 3 days of strength training and 2 days of cardio into your weekly routine'. Now that's a plan that you can track and adjust as necessary.

Self-monitoring is an indispensable tool. You may not always realize when you drift off-course, but by tracking your eating, sleep, and exercise, you'll have tangible data to review. This could be as simple as keeping a food diary or as tech-savvy as wearing a fitness tracker. The reality captured in logs and graphs can be incredibly revealing and can guide your habit refinement.

Build a supportive environment. Surround yourself with people who encourage and support your metamorphosis. Or join a community - whether in-person or online - where members share tips, triumphs, and, yes, even setbacks. Just knowing that you're not navigating this journey alone can amplify your perseverance.

Don't discount the power of a good night's sleep. Quality z's are often the unsung heroes of habit formation. Adequate rest not only energizes you for the day's tasks but also keeps your metabolism and decision-making faculties sharp. Celebrate rest as a pillar of your health, not an obstacle to productivity.

Reward yourself, but think beyond food. Treating yourself to a movie, a massage, or even a new book for hitting milestones reinforces positive behavior without undermining your dietary efforts. Our brains are wired for instant gratification, so these small victories can propel you to the next goal with renewed vigor.

Lastly, practice mindfulness. Being present and aware during meals, work-outs, and even rest can heighten the enjoyment and satisfaction derived from these activities. When you eat, savor each bite; when you move, focus on how your body feels; when resting, really allow yourself to unwind. This level of awareness brings a whole new layer of appreciation to your journey.

Remember, building and sustaining healthy habits isn't a linear process. You'll have peaks and valleys, moments of inspiration, and times of strug-gle. But those hurdles aren't the end; they're simply part of the narrative. Each challenge brings an opportunity to learn about your resilience and adaptability and fine-tune your approach. Embracing these experiences, rather than resisting them, can transform your habits from fleeting novel-ties into robust, lifelong patterns.

Armed with these tips and a mindset focused on progress over perfection, you're now equipped to establish and maintain the habits that will fuel your metabolic reset. Here's to making each day a stride towards a healthier, more vibrant you!

The Importance of Consistency

Embarking on the journey of metabolic reset is like crafting a piece of art; it takes time, patience, and most crucially, consistency. While the excitement of starting anew can fuel the initial surge of motivation, it's the consistent, day-by-day actions that carve out the path to lasting change. Imagine your metabolism as a responsive being, learning and adapting to the cues you provide through your daily habits. It's not the grand gestures but rather the quiet diligence of routine that reshapes this metabolic entity.

Think about the habits that constitute your day. Brushing your teeth isn't a Herculean task because you've made it a non-negotiable part of your routine. That's the level of automaticity you're aiming for with your metabolic habits. It's about reaching a point where healthy choices aren't a source of internal debate; they're simply what you do. Consistency ensures that these behaviors become deeply ingrained, transforming effort into ease over time.

Now, here's a nugget of truth; slight deviations won't capsize your progress. After all, life's unpredictable nature demands flexibility. But when those deviations become the norm—think missing several workouts in a row or letting one indulgent meal turn into a week of poor choices—that's when the ship steers off course. Consistent adherence to your goals doesn't demand perfection, but it does call for a steady hand on the rudder.

Remember, every choice feeds into a feedback loop. Regular exercise, balanced nutrition, and adequate sleep create a symphony of signals to your body, harmonizing your hormones and tuning your metabolism. Miss a beat too often, and the melody of metabolic health can become discordant. The more consistently you maintain these habits, the stronger and more resilient your metabolic system becomes, better able to withstand the odd disruption.

Furthermore, consider the psychological impact of consistency. Each day you align your actions with your goals, you reinforce your identity as someone who takes care of your body and values health and well-being. This self-perception is incredibly powerful, bolstering your belief in your ability to effect change and maintain it.

But let's talk tactics. One key strategy in ensuring consistency is planning. Setbacks often occur when you're caught unprepared. By planning your meals, scheduling your workouts, and carving out time for adequate rest in advance, you're setting yourself up for success. Those plans then act as a contract with yourself, a commitment to the consistency that stands between you and your goals.

Accountability is another potent tool. Sharing your goals with a friend, joining a supportive community, or even maintaining a personal journal can keep you in check. When you know you'll be answering to someone—or even to your future self—you're more likely to stay the course.

It's also worth celebrating the small wins. Acknowledging and rewarding yourself for consistent behavior fosters a sense of progression and keeps the journey enjoyable. Those little victories add up, each one a brick in the foundation of your transformed metabolic health.

Finally, if you slip, don't slide. A lapse in consistency is an opportunity to learn, not a cue to give up. Understand what led to the break in your routine, adjust your strategy, and step back into the rhythm. Resilience is born from these moments, and it's a vital companion on your path to sustainable health.

In a world eager for quick fixes and instant gratification, embracing consistency in your metabolic reset declares a powerful message to yourself and to the world that you're playing the long game. Success isn't a point you reach; it's a manner of traveling. And with steadfast consistency, every step you take is a step toward the vibrant health and vitality you deserve.

Chapter 16

Customizing Your
Metabolic Reset Plan

After arming yourself with knowledge about the fundamentals of metabolism, the building blocks of nutrition, and the profound impact of lifestyle choices, it's time to tailor this wisdom to your unique journey. This isn't a one-size-fits-all scenario; your body's needs are as individual as your fingerprint. In this pivotal chapter, we'll guide you through the nuances of *personalizing your approach* for a metabolic makeover that gels with your realities—not just the ideal scenarios painted in glossy magazines. We'll consider how to navigate the complexities of unique health conditions that may require special attention, underscoring the importance of integrating professional medical insight when necessary. And recognizing that professionals can be crucial allies, this chapter delves into the benefits of working with health professionals to refine your plan, ensuring that every bit of advice is attuned to the symphony of your body's needs. Let's sculpt this framework for metabolic rejuvenation into a masterpiece of health that reverberates with the harmony of individualization.

Personalizing Your Approach

Let's get one thing straight: when it comes to tailoring your metabolic reset plan, there's no one-size-fits-all blueprint. The previous chapters have laid the foundation, but now it's time for the real artistry—sculpting a strategy that fits you like a glove. Your body's unique nuances demand attention, and that's exactly what we'll give them here.

First up, consider your daily routine and lifestyle—these will be your guiding stars. Are you an early riser, powering through meetings by 10 am, or does your energy peak later in the day? Your internal clock, or circadian rhythm, can significantly influence how your body responds to meals and physical activity. Aligning your metabolic plan with your natural cycle can amplify results and make your routine feel almost effortless

Next, let's talk diet, but not in the way you might be accustomed to. Rather than prescribing a rigid menu, think about the foods that make you feel energized and satiated. Food preferences and intolerances play a pivotal role; after all, if you're dreading or reacting poorly to every meal, what's the point? Craft a meal plan that's as enjoyable as it is nourishing. Play with spices, textures, and colors. Make your taste buds your allies in this metabolic venture.

As for intermittent fasting, which we've explored, you'll need to pick a method that syncs with your life. If skipping breakfast leaves you hungry and distracted, perhaps an early window is your best bet. Conversely, if evenings are when you unwind with a meal, then a later eating window might suit you better. Fasting isn't about deprivation—it's about finding a rhythm that enhances your life.

Exercise is another cornerstone of a tailored metabolic reset. Some thrive with the adrenaline rush of high-intensity interval training, while others find solace in the steady cadence of a jog or the quiet focus of strength training. You must find a form of movement that not only ignites your metabolism but also sparks joy. And remember, variety is not just the spice of life—it can prevent plateaus and keep your body guessing.

But it's not just about what you eat and how you move. The unseen players, like hormones and stress, can't be ignored. Chronic stress can wreak havoc on your metabolic goals by stirring up all sorts of hormonal chaos. Finding effective stress management techniques, whether it's meditation, yoga, or a simple breathing exercise, can be as crucial as any diet or workout plan.

Personalization extends far beyond the physical, tapping into the psychological components of habit formation. It's important to know what drives you, what habits are sustainable for you, and most importantly, what makes you fall off the wagon. Forewarned is forearmed, so by anticipating challenges and having strategies ready, you're setting the stage for success.

Let's not forget that life isn't lived in isolation. Whether it's dietary restrictions, medical conditions, or personal goals, you've got to factor these into your blueprint. And when in doubt, enlist the experts. Working with health professionals can help translate the complex symphony of your body's needs into a concrete, achievable plan.

As you continue refining your approach, keep one eye on the mirror and the other on your goal. Reflect on how changes make you feel, and adjust accordingly. Feeling fatigued or irritable? Perhaps tweak your carb intake or shuffle your meal timings. Is your body feeling great, but your mind foggy? Check your hydration or sleep quality. Your body is always communicating; make sure you're listening.

In the end, personalizing your approach is all about becoming fluent in the language of your own body. It's about embracing that your path to a metabolic reset will be uniquely yours. By paying attention to your body's cues and being flexible in your strategy, you're not just embarking on a metabolic reset—you're signing up for a profound journey of self-discovery.

Remember, it's about progress, not perfection. Celebrate the small victories, learn from each step, and fine-tune as you go. Your optimized, personalized metabolic plan isn't just a list of recommendations—it's a living document of your dedication to a healthier you. Let's get that metabolism humming, shall we?

Addressing Unique Health Conditions

As we navigate the process of customizing your metabolic reset plan, it's crucial to acknowledge that there isn't a one-size-fits-all solution, especially when unique health conditions enter the picture. Individual health issues can profoundly impact your metabolism and, consequently, your weight loss journey, which is why your plan needs to be as unique as your DNA.

First things first, let's face it: you might be grappling with health conditions like hypothyroidism or PCOS, which are notorious for putting a wrench in metabolic rates. If this is the case, your approach to resetting your metabolism needs to be tweaked to accommodate these conditions. It's not just about cutting calories; it's about understanding how these conditions interact with your metabolism and responding accordingly.

For those with thyroid problems, the importance of regular check-ups can't be overstressed. The thyroid hormone affects every cell in your body and can make or break your metabolic rate. Your reset plan should sync up with your treatment—this could mean adjusting your iodine intake or finding the perfect spot for selenium-rich foods on your plate.

Now, let's talk about the blood sugar rollercoaster. Conditions like diabetes or insulin resistance require a masterful balancing act of carbs and insulin. Here's where it gets personal—your carb tolerance isn't the same as the next person's. While some can handle complex carbs in moderate amounts, others might need to cozy up to a low-carb plan. And yes, this has huge implications for your weight loss efforts.

And then there's inflammation, often the silent saboteur behind a sluggish metabolism. If you're dealing with an inflammatory condition such as rheumatoid arthritis or IBS, your meal plan can't ignore this. Anti-inflammatory foods like omega-3-rich fish and leafy greens aren't just buzzwords; they could be the key players in your metabolic reboot.

But it's not all about what you can't eat; let's zero in on what you can. If you're living with a health condition, it's essential to lean into foods that work with your body. Whether it's incorporating more plant-based meals for heart health or increasing lean protein to support muscle maintenance for those with sarcopenia, choices matter. Tailoring your diet to your individual needs isn't just smart; it's vital for successful metabolic recalibration.

Beyond food, let's also consider the role of exercise. Depending on your health condition, the dream team of cardio and strength training might need to be modified. For instance, those with joint issues might fare better with low-impact activities like swimming or cycling, which can boost metabolism without the added stress on the body.

For those wondering where to begin, a bit of guidance goes a long way. Collaborating with healthcare professionals—think endocrinologists, nutritionists, and personal trainers—isn't an admission of defeat. It's a strategic move to uncover the intricacies of your health condition and its interaction with your metabolic rate.

Remember, the medication that you're currently taking could also affect your metabolism. Certain drugs can impede weight loss or, on the flip side, increase your appetite. Your doctor can help you weigh the risks and benefits and adjust your plan or medications as needed for your overall health and weight loss goals.

Paying attention to your body's cues is also non-negotiable. If something in your plan doesn't feel right, or if new symptoms emerge, it's important to loop in your doctor. Adjustments to your plan might be necessary, and that's okay—it's all part of personalizing this journey for your body's needs.

In essence, understanding your unique health landscape and responding with a tailored approach is the backbone of your metabolic reset. Nutrition, exercise, and medical support must work together in harmony to navigate the complexities of your health conditions. By doing so, you can not only reset your metabolism but also improve your overall well-being and inch closer to achieving those weight loss goals.

Working with Health Professionals

Embarking on your metabolic reset isn't a journey you have to take alone. In fact, you shouldn't. Working closely with health professionals can significantly enhance your experience and increase your chances of success. These experts serve as allies in your mission, providing essential guidance, personalized advice, and support that cater to your unique health profile.

First and foremost, consider a visit to a registered dietitian specializing in metabolic health. They're trained to understand the intricate dance of nutrition and metabolism. Your dietitian will assess your eating habits, make recommendations based on your dietary needs, and help you plan meals that support your metabolic goals without sacrificing flavor or satisfaction.

Endocrinologists also play a pivotal role if you're dealing with hormonal imbalances that impact metabolism, such as thyroid issues. They can conduct tests, interpret results, and suggest medication or lifestyle changes necessary to correct any imbalances. Sometimes, the difference between a sluggish and a vibrant metabolism lies in the fine-tuning of hormones.

Don't overlook the value of a knowledgeable personal trainer. While they can't prescribe diets or diagnose conditions, personal trainers excel in crafting exercise regimens that dovetail with your metabolic objectives. They'll show you how to achieve the perfect balance between cardiovascular workouts and strength training to rev up your metabolic engine.

For those with specific medical conditions or weight issues, a bariatric physician or weight-loss specialist can offer robust expertise. They understand the complex relationship between weight and metabolism and can help navigate through safe, effective weight loss strategies while monitoring for any medical complications.

Naturopathic doctors, who take a more holistic approach, can also contribute valuable input, especially if you're interested in exploring natural supplements or alternative therapies to complement your metabolic reset. Their broad perspective can shine a light on areas that conventional medicine might overlook.

Remember, regular check-ups with your general practitioner are invaluable for keeping tabs on your overall health throughout this process. They'll keep a vigilant eye on vital signs and blood work to ensure the metabolic changes you're undergoing don't put undue stress on your body's systems.

Also, don't hesitate to seek out a mental health professional if you're finding the psychological aspects of your metabolic reset challenging. A therapist skilled in behavioral change can be instrumental in helping you maintain motivation and manage any emotional hurdles that arise.

Integrating regular consultations with these professionals into your plan isn't just smart; it's essential. Take their feedback seriously, communicate openly about your experiences, and remember that they are there to support you. The collaborative effort will not only aid in tailoring a plan that fits like a glove but also empowers you to make informed decisions about your health.

Finally, as you work with various health professionals, keep a detailed log of their advice, your body's responses, and any adjustments made along the way. This record will be an invaluable reference for both you and your health team as you fine-tune your metabolic reset to perfection.

Better health is within reach, and with the right team by your side, it's a goal that's not only realistic but achievable. Embrace the expertise of health professionals and let their guidance illuminate your path to a renewed, revved-up metabolism.

Chapter 17

Success Stories and Inspirations

As we turn the page to "Success Stories and Inspirations", we immerse ourselves in the powerful narratives of those who've triumphantly navigated the challenges of resetting their metabolism. These are not just tales of pounds shed and clothes sizes dropped; they're profound journeys of individuals reclaiming their vitality, achieving what once felt unattainable. The stories you'll discover here illuminate the path walked by real-life warriors, whose victories over a sluggish metabolism resonate with hard-earned wisdom and tenacity. Through their reflections, we uncover nuggets of practical advice and the undying spark of motivation needed to embark on our metabolic transformation. These portraits of perseverance don't just serve as a testament to what's possible; they light a fire in our bellies, reminding us that our goals are within reach should we approach our metabolic reset with courage, informed strategy, and unyielding resolve.

Real-Life Metabolic Transformation

After learning the fundamentals of metabolism and the importance of nutritional factors, it's exhilarating to see how real-life metabolic transformations can manifest. Let's delve into some inspiring tales of those who've turned their metabolic health around with dedication, education, and a sprinkle of hard work.

Consider James, a man in his mid-40s who felt trapped by a sluggish metabolism. Despite routine exercise, he couldn't shake off those extra pounds. James's breakthrough came when he embraced a holistic approach, tweaking his diet to favor whole foods while incorporating intermittent fasting. The weight began to melt away, and his energy levels skyrocketed, illustrating the power of syncing lifestyle with metabolic needs.

Then there's Maria, a woman who not only struggled with weight but also with persistent fatigue and brain fog. She honed in on her sleep patterns, realizing that her metabolism was in cahoots with her circadian rhythm. By establishing a routine, focusing on sleep hygiene, and managing her stress, Maria's cognitive function improved, and her metabolic rate increased, proving the substantial impact of sleep on our metabolic engines.

Stories like these are galvanizing, yes? They underscore that it's never too late to influence your metabolic health. It's essential to recognize that metabolism isn't merely about burning calories; it's about how your body employs energy — a concept Robert, a retired veteran, took to heart. Integrating strength training into his regimen, he overturned years of metabolic decline. His muscles became more efficient at using energy, and his metabolic age began to defy his chronological years.

Some transformations are even more profound. Take Lisa, whose diet was once laden with processed sugars, contributing to a rollercoaster of blood sugar spikes and crashes. Upon learning the intrinsic link between balanced blood sugar and a robust metabolism, Lisa incrementally reduced her intake of simple carbs. In their stead, she introduced fiber-rich foods, which sent her metabolism into a newfound harmony and unlocked weight loss that had once seemed implausible.

Consider how these transformations exhibit the impact of personalized metabolic interventions. No one-size-fits-all solution exists when it comes to resetting your metabolism. Yet, there's something profound in the way these individuals harnessed their unique situations to breathe life into their metabolic health.

What these vignettes also reveal is the power of patience and persistence. Many people embark on this journey expecting quick results, but the truth is that metabolic reset is a process. It involves unraveling habits that may have entrenched themselves over decades and rediscovering a balance that resonates with your body's natural rhythms.

An essential takeaway from these success stories is the role of self-awareness. By keeping tabs on their reactions to various dietary and lifestyle changes, these individuals could tailor their approaches to suit their evolving needs. It wasn't a straightforward path, and there were surely bumps along the road, but with each small victory, their resolve was steeled, and their metabolic health was reinforced.

So, what can you glean from these stories for your journey? These aren't merely weight loss narratives; they're chronicles of individuals claiming agency over their health. They teach us that with the right information, tools, and mindset, a metabolic overhaul is within your grasp, and the outcomes can extend far beyond the scale, encompassing a complete renaissance of vitality and well-being.

Take these anecdotes as a beacon of possibility for your metabolic reset — a clear indication that transformation is tangible. They don't suggest a magical or abrupt overhaul but rather the rewards that await on the other side of consistent, mindful efforts. Embrace these lessons and let them fuel your path to a revitalized metabolism and a life of vibrancy.

As we turn the page to explore further, remember these tales of transformation. Allow them to kindle a fire of inspiration within you, one that will illuminate the steps of your own metabolic journey. As for the specifics on how these individuals made such remarkable changes — we will delve deeper into that as we pivot to the next sections, leaving you equipped to chart a path towards your personalized metabolic nirvana.

Lessons Learned from Success Stories

Diving into the vortex of success stories, there's a trove of insights waiting to be unearthed. Men and women who've successfully reset their metabolism and shed pounds often share a few critical elements that are pivotal in shaping their journey. These elements become the compass for those still navigating the path of metabolic transformation.

A recurring theme is the unabashed embrace of education. Those who take the time to understand the intricate dance of hormones and nutrients within their body tend to fare better. It's not just about what you eat, but also understanding how your body uses it. This knowledge empowers individuals to make informed decisions rather than following diet trends blindly.

Consistency is the thread weaving through each success narrative. Implementing small, sustainable changes consistently over time has proven more fruitful than drastic overhauls that fizzle out. It's like building a fortress brick by brick—strength lies not in quickness but in the steadfast layering of habits.

Speaking of habits, customization is also key. What works for one person might be another's downfall. The successful metabolically transformed individuals often recount the importance of tailoring their diet and exercise routines to fit their unique lifestyles, needs, and preferences. They remind us that a one-size-fits-all approach rarely sizes up.

Flexibility, both in mindset and method, emerges as another cornerstone. Successful individuals don't crumble in the face of a setback; they adapt. Whether it's tweaking a meal plan, modifying a workout, or even overcoming a weight loss plateau, the ability to pivot and persist highlights a lesson in resilience.

Intertwined with flexibility is the practice of mindfulness—both in eating and living. Being mentally present for each meal, savoring the flavors, and listening to the body's cues for fullness and satisfaction is often mentioned as a transformational experience. The mindfulness extends beyond the plate, fostering a deeper connection with oneself and the journey.

Another observation is the power of community. No man is an island, and indeed, no weight loss journey thrives in isolation. Those who have found success often credit support systems, whether online forums, fitness groups, or understanding families, for providing motivation and accountability.

It's impossible to overlook the influence of sleep and stress management. Time and again, success stories illustrate how prioritizing sleep and finding effective ways to destress have positively impacted their metabolic health. In a world that often prides itself on hustle and bustle, they've learned that rest and relaxation aren't just luxuries; they're necessities.

The significance of tracking progress with tangible metrics also surfaces in these tales of triumph. Whether through journaling, apps, or wearable devices, monitoring growth has sparked motivation and provided clear indications of when to celebrate victories or recalibrate strategies.

Last but not least, successful individuals often preach the doctrine of patience. Metabolic reset is not an instant makeover; it's a progressive journey. They encourage embracing the slow, steady progress and viewing it not as a race, but as a lifelong investment in health and wellbeing.

Each lesson learned is a beacon for those still fighting the good fight. They are testaments to the triumph of spirit over circumstance, and an affirmation that with the right mindset, tools, and persistence, resetting your metabolism and achieving health goals is within reach.

Using Inspiration for Your Journey

As we've delved deep into the complexities of metabolism and the myriad strategies to reset it, we reach a pivotal point in our journey—the fuel that drives our motivation. Harnessing inspiration can be as crucial as understanding the science behind metabolic health. In this section, we'll explore how to use the power of real-life success stories to bolster your resolve and keep your metabolic aspirations burning bright.

It's undeniable that hearing about others who've triumphed over similar struggles has an encouraging effect. So, let's pull that power into our orbit. Dive into the narratives of men and women who've transformed their metabolic health and, in doing so, redefined their lives. The beauty lies not in mirroring their paths, but in sifting through their experiences to discover kindling for your fire.

Remember that every success story starts with a single step, often in challenging circumstances. Whether it's the tale of a busy parent finding time to prioritize their health, or an individual overcoming a lifelong battle with weight management, these stories echo a resounding theme—you can do it, too. Reflect on their commitment and the adaptations they made along the way, and consider how you could apply the lessons they learned to your unique situation.

Many have found solace and strength in the midst of frustration, with periods where progress stalls, known as plateaus. Their stories reveal the reality that setbacks are simply part of the process, not the end of the road. By learning how they pushed through these times, you can arm yourself with an arsenal of strategies to confront your own plateau should you encounter one.

As you absorb these tales, focus on the strategies that resonate with your lifestyle. Maybe it's the way someone integrated intermittent fasting into a hectic schedule, or perhaps the inventive meal planning that transformed another's nutritional intake. These practical takeaways are golden nuggets you can weave into the fabric of your life.

It's also essential to note the mental shifts that come with profound physical change. Success stories often highlight the importance of a positive mindset, the willingness to adapt, and steadfastness in the face of adversity. The mental metamorphosis is as impactful as the physical—one cannot exist without the other. Let the psychological resilience exhibited by these individuals inspire a mental fortitude you can call upon when needed.

Importantly, don't just read these stories—engage with them. Jot down thoughts, underline passages that strike a chord, or take notes on strategies that seem particularly beneficial. This active engagement helps transform passive reading into active inspiration. Over time, you'll compile a personal treasury of motivational mantras and tricks tailored to keep your journey alive.

Consider starting a journal to reflect on these inspirations and how they can blend into your metabolic reset. As you mark your progress, revisit your journal. This will serve as a vivid reminder of not just where you've been but the collective wisdom that's been imparted to you by those who've walked this path before.

Lastly, remember the potency of sharing your successes, both big and small. As you make strides in your metabolic journey, your narrative may become a beacon for others. The inspiration is cyclical—the stories that propel you forward will be joined by your own, completing a circle of motivation that stretches far beyond a single individual.

The journey towards resetting your metabolism and forging a healthier life is not one you tread alone. Let the inspiration of others who've reached their destination serve as lighthouses guiding you through challenging waters. With each success story, allow a spark of possibility to ignite within you, and let it be the light that leads you through your journey of transformation.

Chapter 18

The Challenge of Eating Out and Social Events

Navigating the tantalizing menus of restaurants or the appetizing spreads at social gatherings poses a unique challenge when you're revved up to reset your metabolism. It's the tug-of-war between the pleasure of the palate and the goals for your waistline where many find themselves in a pickle. You're not just eating for sustenance; it's also about pleasure, celebration, and community. And let's be real, that slice of cheesecake or the creamy carbonara is singing your name. But hold on, there are proven strategies to help you stay the course without feeling like you're skimping on the joys of life. It's about smart choices, not just what's on your plate, but how you approach the whole scenario—small portions, mindful eating, and balanced indulgence can be your allies. Let's peel back the layers of this common conundrum, revealing that lasting weight loss and enjoying social meals aren't mutually exclusive. With the right mindset, you can savor the conviviality without halting your metabolic momentum.

How to Stay on Track When Dining Out

Eating out is a delightful indulgence and a cornerstone of social interactions. Still, when you're in the process of resetting your metabolism and aiming for weight loss, it can present certain challenges. Fear not; with a strategic game plan, you can still enjoy the pleasures of dining out without derailing your goals. Let's dive into actionable tips that align with your metabolic reset and allow you to stay on track even when you're not the one controlling the stove.

First things first, before stepping out, become a menu mastermind. Most restaurants now provide their menus online. Use this to your advantage by perusing the options in advance and deciding what to order. That way, you won't be swayed by the alluring descriptions or others' choices once you're there. Pick dishes that are rich in lean proteins, contain healthy fats, and are filled with vegetables—the trifecta for keeping your metabolism ticking.

Adopt the art of customization. It's easy to assume that menu items are set in stone, but chefs are typically more than willing to accommodate modifications. Ask for dressings and sauces on the side, swap out starchy sides for extra veggies, or request that your meal be cooked with less oil or butter. These tweaks might seem minor, but they add up in the long run, enabling you to stay within the parameters of your metabolic reset plan.

Don't arrive ravenous. The hungrier you are, the more likely you are to make decisions driven by cravings rather than health goals. Have a healthy snack like a small handful of nuts or a piece of fruit before you head out. This can curb your appetite and help you resist the breadbasket's siren call—putting you in control from the start.

Hydration is your hidden ally when dining out. Not only does it help your metabolic function, but sipping on water throughout your meal can slow down your eating pace and help you feel fuller faster. Aim to drink a glass of water before your meal arrives, and continue to hydrate as you eat. Steer clear of calorie-dense drinks such as sodas or sugary cocktails, which can be an unexpected caloric downfall.

The power of portion control cannot be overemphasized. Restaurant servings are notoriously oversized. Rather than trying to finish everything on your plate, mentally note what an appropriate serving looks like based on your dietary plan. Eat until you're satisfied, not stuffed, and ask for a to-go box for leftovers. This not only helps you spread the calorie intake but also turns one meal into two.

Eating slowly is more than just good manners; it allows your body time to recognize fullness. Our metabolism and the signals that indicate satiety are not instantaneous. By putting your cutlery down between bites and engaging in conversation, you give your body the time to process the food and signal when it's time to stop.

Remember to consider the context of your entire day. If you know you'll be dining out in the evening, plan your earlier meals accordingly. Lighter meals packed with fiber will help you maintain stable blood sugar levels throughout the day and make it easier to keep your dinner within reasonable limits.

Beware of the after-meal enticements; just because you navigated dinner doesn't mean the battle's won. Desserts and after-dinner drinks carry a hefty caloric punch and often contain refined sugars that can spike your blood sugar. If you must indulge, share dessert with others at the table to satisfy the sweet tooth while keeping portions in check.

Lastly, maintain perspective. A single meal out is just one of many, and it's the overall pattern of eating that matters most for your metabolic health. If a meal doesn't go as planned, don't beat yourself up. Acknowledge it as an isolated incident and return to your well-structured plan with your next meal. Eating out should be enjoyable, not anxiety-inducing. Part of creating a sustainable, healthy lifestyle is being able to adapt without guilt.

In conclusion, dining out doesn't have to derail your dietary goals. With a little planning and strategy, you can enjoy the social and culinary delights that restaurants offer while keeping your metabolic reset on course. Be proactive, stay mindful, and savor not only the food but the success of managing your goals in any setting.

Strategies for Managing Social Eating

Embarking on a journey to reset your metabolism while facing a social calendar dotted with dining out and events might seem daunting. It's common to feel like your goals and social life are at odds, but trust me, they don't have to be. With the right strategies, you can navigate these settings without derailing your progress. In this section, we'll explore how to maintain your metabolic focus amid the inevitable social gatherings that involve food and drink.

First and foremost, planning is your strongest ally. Before attending any event, familiarize yourself with the menu or ask your host about the meal options. Going in with a planned idea of what you can eat allows you to focus on socializing instead of stressing over food choices. When possible, opt for dishes that emphasize proteins and vegetables, which support your metabolism and help you feel full longer.

Perhaps the environment doesn't offer the most metabolic-friendly options; this is where portion control becomes your superpower. Allowing yourself to enjoy a small serving of something indulgent can satisfy cravings and prevent the feeling of deprivation. Remember, it's about finding a balance that works for you. Portion control isn't about scarcity; it's about empowerment — the power to choose and still align with your goals.

Drinks, like food, can be full of hidden sugars and empty calories that disrupt metabolic balance. An alternative is to infuse your gatherings with sparkling water, a twist of citrus, or a splash of juice for a refreshing and metabolism-friendly toast. And if you do decide to enjoy an alcoholic beverage, moderation is key. Pair it with plenty of water to stay hydrated and keep your system in check.

When eating in a group setting, pacing yourself can make all the difference. Don't feel compelled to keep up with the eating speed of others. Instead, eat slowly and savor your food—this can also help regulate the amount you consume and give your body the time it needs to signal fullness.

But what about those moments when you're just not sure what will be served? That's where a pre-event snack comes in handy. Enjoying a nutritious snack before you head out can curb hunger and provide you with the fortitude to make mindful choices, rather than succumbing to whatever's available because you're ravenous.

Don't underestimate the power of saying 'no.' While it might seem uncomfortable at first, setting boundaries is a necessary part of maintaining a lifestyle that supports your metabolic goals. You're not obligated to taste everything that's offered to you. Politely declining with a smile is a skill worth mastering, and it gets easier with practice.

Communication is also an essential tool. Share your health goals with friends and family. Open conversations can lead to understanding, and they'll likely want to support your journey. They may even adjust their menu or venue choice to accommodate your needs. You might even inspire them to make healthier choices too!

Lastly, always keep in mind that one meal or one event won't make or break your progress. If you do indulge more than intended, it's not the end of your metabolic reset. What matters most is getting back on track with the next meal. Consistency over time is what brings about change, not perfection in a single evening.

With these strategies in play, social eating becomes less about anxiety and more about the joy of sharing experiences with others while staying true to your aims. Enjoy your social life and your metabolic-reset journey simultaneously, because balance is not only possible—it's sustainable.

Remember, you're rewriting your story, one meal, one event at a time. Social eating doesn't have to be a challenge; it can be an opportunity to practice resilience and flexibility within your metabolic reset plan. Together, these strategies fortify your commitment to yourself and your health, ensuring that your social engagements enrich rather than hinder your progress.

Dealing with Peer Pressure

So you've braved the restaurant menus and navigated the buffet table with success—your metabolic reset journey is well on its way. But what happens when we run into the subtle, yet powerful force known as peer pressure? It's a common roadblock, one that can derail even the most dedicated health enthusiast. Let's dive in and unpack some strategies to keep you steady when the social seas get turbulent.

First things first, remember this: you're in control. Your dietary choices are personal, and they play a pivotal role in resetting your metabolism. When friends, coworkers, or family members coax you to "just have one bite," it's crucial to stand your ground firmly but politely. A simple "No, thank you" often suffices, but if pressed further, a brief explanation that you're focusing on your health and specific food choices can be highly effective. Effective communication is your shield against the advances of persuasive pals.

Now, let's approach this with some savvy. Before heading out, consider informing your host or friends about your dietary needs. This preemptive strike can often cool the fires of peer pressure before they even spark. By setting the stage early, you establish a mutual understanding that may encourage them to support rather than challenge your resolve.

If the spotlight gets too hot, flip the script. Accentuate the positive by expressing the benefits you've experienced since undertaking this metamorphic health journey. People get intrigued by progress, and this could make the focus of the conversation your success, instead of what's on or absent from your plate. Inspiring others is a nice side-effect, don't you think?

Then there's the buddy system. Bring along a friend who's also committed to healthy eating or is supportive of your metabolic goals. There's strength in numbers, and having an ally at the dinner table can help diffuse the pressure from the group.

Choosing to abstain from certain foods or beverages can sometimes provoke unwelcome attention, leading to that dreaded pressure. Be proactive with your choices; seek out menu options that fit your metabolic reset plan and suggest restaurants that offer a variety of suitable dishes. This way, you can indulge in the social atmosphere without compromising your progress.

What about those special occasions—birthdays, weddings, or holidays? These situations can be particularly challenging. A helpful tip is to eat something before the event. Heading out on a full stomach can minimize the temptation to stray from your eating plan when high-pressure social feasting starts.

Steadfast yet struggling? Turn to visualization techniques. Imagine the after-effects of giving in to peer pressure—the disharmony in your metabolic progress, the lingering regret. Now contrast that with the pride of sticking to your plan. By foreseeing the outcomes of your choices, the right decision becomes clearer, and your willpower is galvanized.

It's also essential to forgive yourself should you succumb to the occasional slip. This journey is not about perfection; it's about consistency and learning. Use any missteps as learning opportunities to strengthen your resolve for the next time you're in a similar situation.

Lastly, don't overlook the influence of non-verbal cues. Holding a glass of water or keeping your plate partially filled can deter the food-pushers and signal that you're content. These subtle signals can deflect attention without needing to voice your decline over and over.

Peer pressure is a natural element of social dining, but it doesn't have to dictate your dietary decisions. Remember why you started this metabolic reset in the first place—your health. Armed with these strategies, you're well-equipped to maintain your course and enjoy the socializing without jeopardizing your progress. Onward and upward!

Chapter 19

Common Pitfalls to Avoid

As we've dissected the elements of a successful metabolic reset—balancing blood sugar, the synergy between gut health and metabolism, and the potent influence of sleep—it's crucial to pivot our attention to the common pitfalls that can easily derail our efforts. Missteps like reaching for quick fixes that promise rapid weight loss can lead to metabolic mayhem rather than health. These solutions often lack the nutritional foundation your body craves and can leave you feeling unsatisfied, only to see the pounds creep back on. Then there's the allure of fad diets—sure, they're trendy and pervasive in media, but they tend to swing you from one extreme to another, setting you up for a cringe-worthy rebound. And let's not forget the mental game; overcoming setbacks is about more than willpower; it's about equipping yourself with the strategies to bounce back stronger, without letting old habits cut your journey short. Being mindful of these pitfalls and approaching your metabolic reset with a keen eye will steer you clear of these traps and keep you on the path toward sustainable weight loss and optimal well-being.

Recognizing and Overcoming Obstacles

As we transition from understanding what to avoid, let's zone in on the challenges you may face and how to redefine them as opportunities to strengthen your resolve. First off, obstacles in resetting your metabolism aren't failures; they're signs that you're pushing boundaries and stepping out of your comfort zone. It's normal to hit a few bumps on this journey. The aim here isn't to glide through without effort but to learn to navigate and eventually master the rough waters of metabolic change!

Ever start a diet or workout plan with fire, only to have it fizzle out in the face of a hurdle? That's an incredibly common experience. Frustration is as much a part of metabolic reset as is the joy of seeing results. When you notice your enthusiasm waning after, say, a holiday weekend filled with indulgence, relax. Acknowledge that there will be days when the plan goes awry. Embrace them. These are the moments that build resilience. Then, redirect your focus and remember why you started. Your goals aren't tied to a single slip-up; they're built on a consistent, long-term approach.

It's easy to underestimate how much mental bandwidth managing your metabolic health requires. You're changing habits that have been ingrained for years, perhaps even decades. If you find yourself forgetting or skipping parts of your reset plan, don't throw in the towel. Instead, look at your routine: Is it too complex? Are there ways to simplify or integrate it more seamlessly into your life? Simplification isn't admitting defeat; it's designing a sustainable approach that works for you.

Another speed bump people often encounter is plateaus. They are not a dead end but rather a sign that your body's adapting. This adaptation is fascinating evidence of your body's intelligence, but it can be maddening when the scale won't budge. The key here is to tweak your routine—add variety to your diet, change up your exercise regimen, or ensure you're getting enough sleep and managing stress.

Stress—yes, let's talk about that saboteur. It can wreak havoc on your metabolism and just about every other aspect of your health. It raises cortisol levels, which can impede weight loss and harm your overall well-being. It's vital to incorporate stress-reduction techniques like meditation, deep-breathing exercises, or even just a daily walk in nature. These practices aren't just feel-good activities; they directly combat cortisol and help keep your metabolic reset on track.

Lapses in motivation can be another significant obstacle. Here's where setting up a support system can be a game-changer. Whether it's a workout buddy, an online support group, or a healthcare professional, having someone to share the journey with can make all the difference. They can provide a simultaneous source of motivation and accountability—two essential ingredients for overcoming those moments when going it alone feels too tough.

On the topic of tough moments, remember the adage about the best-laid plans? Well, life can sometimes throw you a curveball, be it an illness, a personal loss, or an overwhelming work deadline. These experiences can temporarily derail your metabolic reset. When they happen, practice self-compassion rather than self-punishment. Take the time you need to deal with what's important and return to your plan when you're ready. Tenacity isn't measured by never falling; it's about how many times you get back up.

Then there's the influence of our digital age—info overload. It's easy to get caught up in contrasting advice and the latest trends promising quick results. Stay rooted in evidence-based practices and don't jump ship every time a new "miracle cure" appears on your newsfeed. Consistency in the right habits is what leads to success, not jumping from one quick fix to another.

Hunger and cravings can certainly throw a wrench in the works. When they strike, reflect on the cause. Are you genuinely hungry, or are you potentially thirsty, bored, or dealing with emotional hunger instead? Understanding the root of your cravings can detour you away from unnecessary snacking and help keep your metabolic reset journey on course.

Recall that every obstacle is a teacher in disguise, ready to instruct you on the subtle art of listening to your body and persevering with purpose. By overcoming each challenge, you're not just closer to your goal weight or a more effervescent energy level. You're also mastering the ability to confront and conquer the many obstacles that life inevitably throws your way. That's a skill that will serve you far beyond the numbers on the scale.

Avoiding Quick Fixes and Fad Diets

We've just navigated through the myriad ways to support our bodies in resetting their metabolism, but there's a siren song that can easily lead us astray: the allure of quick fixes and fad diets. They tempt us with promises of rapid weight loss and effortless results, targeting our desires for immediate gratification. But let's get real - these superficial solutions are usually fraught with drawbacks that can hinder our long-term metabolic health.

Fad diets often come with flashy names and celebrity endorsements, making them hard to resist. They might tell you to shun certain food groups or to gulp down specially formulated concoctions. However, one thing they consistently lack is sustainability. They aren't built for the long game, which is what truly resetting your metabolism is all about. These diets may lead to swift weight changes, but often, those pounds come right back, with a few extra friends.

Consider the impact of severe calorie restriction, a common theme in fad dieting. It's like putting your body in economic recession mode; sure, you'll lose weight, but at what cost? Your body isn't getting the resources it needs to function optimally. This can throw your hormones out of whack, and you can bet your metabolism isn't going to thrive in such conditions. Instead, it may slow down further to conserve energy, exactly the opposite of what you're aiming for.

Then there's the psychological toll. Fad diets are notorious for their strict rules and can make you feel guilty about eating 'forbidden' foods. This often leads to an unhealthy relationship with food, where eating becomes a source of stress rather than nourishment. A metabolic reset isn't about demonizing food but learning to understand and appreciate it for the energy and nutrients it provides.

It's also vital to know that these diets don't consider your individuality. What works for one person might not work for you. Your body's unique metabolic needs, lifestyle, preferences, and limitations should guide your dietary choices, not the latest trend sweeping social media. Personalization is key to a successful metabolic transformation.

Fad diets also neglect the importance of a balanced diet, which is crucial for metabolic health. Your body needs a symphony of nutrients working in harmony, not just a solo act. From vitamins and minerals to macronutrients like proteins and healthy fats, all play integral roles in maintaining a robust metabolism.

Beyond the physical aspects, think about the sense of community and shared meals. Fad diets can isolate you, making it hard to participate in social gatherings and family dinners. Is it worth it to lose weight at the expense of enjoying life's pleasures? A balanced approach allows you to indulge in these moments mindfully, without compromising your metabolic goals.

So, how can you spot a fad diet? Watch out for these red flags:

- Unrealistic claims

- A drastic reduction in calorie intake

- Elimination of whole food groups

- A reliance on specific products sold by the promoters

If it sounds too good to be true, it likely is. These diets don't offer the magic bullet they claim to.

Rather than reaching for a quick fix, invest in building healthy, sustainable habits that support your metabolic health in the long run. Embrace a variety of fresh, whole foods, listen to your body's hunger cues, and find joy in physical activities that get your blood pumping. Remember, the goal is a reset—a revival of your body's natural rhythm and functionality, not a temporary patch job.

In conclusion, steer clear of the fad diet trap. They're not just ineffective; they can be detrimental to your overall health. Instead, nourish your body with thoughtful choices that promote metabolic balance. It might not be the quick-fix solution, but it's the foundation for sustainable change and true well-being.

Coping with Setbacks

Life has a funny way of throwing curveballs just when you think you've hit your stride. When working toward a metabolic reset, it's not if but when you'll face setbacks. It might begin with a missed workout or succumbing to a sugary temptation. Suddenly, you might find yourself feeling like you've taken three steps back. Take heart; these moments don't define your journey—they're just part of the process.

First things first, let's agree that perfection is off the table. No one nails their dietary and lifestyle changes 100% of the time, and that's okay. What's essential is learning to bounce back with resilience. When you experience a setback, pause and reflect. What led to this detour? Often, there's an emotional trigger or situational stressor at play. Unpacking what happened can provide valuable insights that help you avoid similar pitfalls in the future.

Keep a flexible mindset. Instead of seeing an indulgent meal as a complete derailment, consider it a single, isolated choice that doesn't automatically erase all your progress. The power lies in the next decision you make. Aim to return to your healthy habits during your next meal or workout session. It's about progression, not perfection.

Deprivation can be a surefire road to relapse. If you're feeling restricted by your diet, it's time to spice up your meal plan. No one can sustain themselves on bland, repetitive foods indefinitely. Explore new recipes, try different spices, and find creative ways to incorporate variety into your dietary routine. Your taste buds—and your metabolism—will thank you for it.

Stress management also plays a crucial role in coping with setbacks. When stressed, our bodies produce cortisol, which can adversely affect our metabolic health. Find stress-reducing techniques that work for you, whether meditation, yoga, or a simple walk outside. Reducing stress can help keep your metabolism in check and lessen the likelihood of comfort eating.

It's also crucial to have a support system. Share your goals with friends, family, or a supportive online community. They can offer encouragement, advice, or a sympathetic ear when needed. Don't underestimate the power of shared experiences; sometimes, knowing others are on a similar path can make all the difference.

Remember, sleep is a secret weapon against setbacks. Ensuring you get enough quality sleep can improve your mood, help regulate appetite hormones, and support metabolic health. Prioritize rest as much as exercise and nutrition; your body needs recovery to function optimally.

Set small, attainable goals to regain your confidence. If a setback has left you feeling overwhelmed, simplify your approach. Instead of focusing on the big picture, set a modest goal for the day or week ahead. Success breeds success, and each small victory can help rebuild your momentum.

Action is an antidote to despair. When facing setbacks, don't let inaction set in. Take proactive steps, no matter how small they seem. Whether that's a 10-minute walk or choosing a salad over fries with your meal, each positive choice sets the stage for more. Action catalyzes further action—use it to your advantage.

In conclusion, setbacks can be humbling, but they're not the end of the world. They're a natural part of the ebb and flow of life's rhythms. Learning to navigate these moments with resilience and grace can transform them from stumbling blocks to stepping stones on your journey to metabolic health. So take a deep breath, recalibrate, and remember that tomorrow is a new day to continue making strides toward your goals.

Chapter 20

Beyond Weight Loss

The Wider Health Benefits of a Metabolic Reset

If you think your metabolic reset is just about shedding those stubborn pounds, you're in for a pleasant surprise. Embarking on this journey does more than whittle your waistline; it profoundly amplifies your overall well-being. Imagine waking up with a vigor you haven't felt since your teenage years; that's the kind of energetic surge we're discussing post-reset. But let's not stop there – clarity of mind becomes the norm, not a caffeine-induced rarity. You'll find yourself sharper, more focused, and ready to tackle complex tasks with newfound ease. And here's the real kicker: by fine-tuning your body's metabolic processes, you're setting the stage for a longer, more disease-resistant life. That's right, this goes beyond the mirror and scale; it's about gifting your future self with the best health prospects imaginable. So, as we dive into the potent ripple effects of a metabolic reset, you'll see it's not just about the numbers—it's about a rejuvenated, vibrant existence that radiates through every facet of your life.

Improved Energy Levels

As we delve into the increased vitality that accompanies a metabolic reset, it's essential to understand that this is more than just about shedding those stubborn pounds. It's an overhaul that recharges your entire system, giving you the capacity not only to lose weight but also to live life with an elevated zest.

Think about it for a moment - energy is the currency of our bodies. When you have more of it, every task seems a bit easier, and every challenge a bit more surmountable. But achieving this isn't just about willing yourself to feel less tired; it's a biological tune-up that begins at the most fundamental level of your body's functioning - your metabolism. When your metabolism resets, it's like upgrading your body's energy factories.

A metabolic reset cranks up the efficiency of your mitochondria, those tiny powerhouses within your cells that convert food and oxygen into energy. It recalibrates your body's use of carbohydrates and fats, optimizing for a sustained release of energy, rather than the short bursts and crashes we often experience after indulging in sugary snacks or processed meals. It's the difference between a roaring fire providing warmth all night and a flashpaper that flares up and extinguishes in an instant.

The harmony between hormones like insulin and glucagon stabilizes after a reset. As they work better together, they choreograph a delicate dance that keeps your blood sugar levels steady. And what does this mean for you? No more mid-afternoon crashes, no more cravings that hijack your attention. It means waking up feeling refreshed, with energy that lasts throughout the day - the kind that's stable, enduring, and reliable.

Moreover, improved hydration and micronutrient intake, which are central to a metabolic reset, play a pivotal role. These elements are akin to oiling the gears of your body's machinery. Adequate hydration ensures that energy-generating reactions occur without a hitch, while vitamins and minerals act as co-factors for enzymes that speed up those very metabolic reactions that keep you vibrant and active.

Intermittent fasting, which often goes hand-in-hand with metabolic resets, can also amplify your energy levels. This practice not only assists in weight loss but also prompts your cells to improve their waste removal processes and repair functions. Consequently, your cells become more proficient at generating energy, which translates to you feeling more awake and alive.

Additionally, as your gut health improves – a facet we can't overlook in a metabolic reset – you'll find that you have more energy. A gut that's functioning optimally absorbs nutrients better, and better nutrient absorption means better energy production. It's like upgrading from a clunky, old steam engine to a sleek, new maglev train.

However, let's not forget exercise, the spark that ignites your metabolic engine. As you incorporate a balanced exercise program, your body's capability to utilize energy efficiently reaches new heights. With increased muscle mass and cardiovascular fitness, your organism becomes a connoisseur of energy management, letting you engage in daily activities with less fatigue.

Remember that the road to improved energy levels isn't an overnight journey. It requires consistent effort in aligning meals, sleep, and lifestyle with the principles of metabolic health. Over time, as you recalibrate, you'll notice the difference. You'll be able to push through that late-afternoon slump, dedicate yourself more wholly to your fitness routine, and find mental clarity where there was once fog.

Just imagine being able to meet the day's demands head-on and still having enough fuel in the tank for an engaging evening with family or an impromptu adventure with friends. That's the true mark of a successful metabolic reset. So, if you've ever wondered if there's a secret to boundless energy, this holistic approach to renewed metabolism is your profound, unequivocal answer.

Enhanced Mental Clarity

As we wade deeper into the multifaceted health perks of a metabolic reset, it's crystal clear that the brain is in for a treat as much as the body is. Let's dive into the profound effect a metabolic overhaul can have on your mental clarity.

Cast your mind back to a day when you felt sharp, focused, and able to tackle the most complex of puzzles with ease. It's not just a nostalgic thought; it's a state of being that hinges on diet, lifestyle, and hormonal balance. By resetting your metabolism, you're indirectly tuning up your brain's engine, leading to noticeably clearer thinking. But how does that work, you may wonder?

When your metabolism is out of whack, it's not just your waistline that bears the brunt—your brain does too. Fluctuating blood sugar caused by a sluggish metabolism can send your mental state on a rollercoaster, leaving you cloudy and unfocused. Consistent energy levels are the golden ticket to bulletproof concentration, and a slapped-together metabolic reset is the competitive edge you need.

Glycogen, our brain's preferred source of energy, arrives on a steady conveyor belt when your metabolism is in top shape. No more mid-afternoon crashes or wandering thoughts—your brain has the continuous fuel it needs to operate at peak efficiency. This even delivery makes for a serene mental environment where cognizance reigns supreme, and the fog of confusion evaporates.

Intermittent fasting, a prime player in metabolic resets, plays its part too. It's been linked to increased production of brain-derived neurotrophic factor (BDNF), a protein that's like brain fertilizer, encouraging new neuron growth and enhancing cognitive functions. Think of it as a personal trainer for your brain, pushing your mental muscles to grow stronger and sharper with every passing day.

Then there's the hormone balance ballet. When you fine-tune your metabolism, insulin sensitivity improves, thyroid function normalizes, and stress hormones like cortisol take a back seat. This harmonious hormone dance translates into a calm, clear state of mind where decisions are made with precision, and thoughts flow like a serene river.

Don't forget about inflammation, the ultimate party crasher. A reset metabolism diminishes systemic inflammation, which can otherwise act like a smog on the brain, clouding judgment and dampening spirits. With the haze lifted, cognitive function can soar to new heights, making room for productivity and creativity to flourish.

Is there anything better than a good night's sleep to grease those cerebral gears? Well, metabolic synchronization leads to better sleep patterns. With sound sleep every night, you're well on your way to a mind that's rested, rejuvenated, and ready to unravel the mysteries of the universe—or at least power through your to-do list.

Moreover, it's not just an immediate boost in mental agility we're talking about; maintaining a healthy metabolism can contribute to long-term brain health. Evidence suggests it may fend off cognitive decline and keep age-related brain fog at bay. It's as if you're investing in a high-performance brain fund for your golden years.

So there you have it—a metabolic reset could be your brain's ally in the battle against fuzziness and forgetfulness. It brings a sense of clarity that illuminates your mental landscape, guiding you to make better choices, think more creatively, and enjoy a sharper, more focused life. And who wouldn't want a slice of that genius pie?

Longevity and Disease Prevention

So, we've waded through the intricacies of a metabolic reset, and we've explored how it ramps up your energy and sharpens your mind, but let's dive into perhaps its most compelling domain: longevity and disease prevention. It's not just about shedding pounds—it's about adding years of quality life!

Starting our discussion with longevity, it's essential to grasp that metabolic health is intricately linked to aging. When your metabolism hums like a well-oiled machine, it doesn't just burn calories efficiently; it also moderates the wear and tear on your body. Less damage means less aging, plain and simple. A metabolic reset is like hitting the rejuvenate button on your body's cellular machinery, which can keep you feeling spry well into your later years.

Moving on to disease prevention, let's get this straight: your metabolism holds the keys to the kingdom of your overall health. Multiple studies have consistently made the connection between metabolic dysfunction and a higher risk of chronic diseases like type 2 diabetes, heart disease, and certain cancers. By resetting your metabolism, you're essentially setting up a defense system against these conditions.

Consider how a stable metabolic rate aids in maintaining balanced blood sugar levels. Steady blood sugar means less stress on your pancreas and less risk of developing insulin resistance—one of the culprits behind type 2 diabetes. Plus, let's not forget that insulin resistance is a gateway for a myriad of other health issues.

Let's also chat about inflammation—often the body's response to excess fat, particularly the visceral kind that likes to wrap itself around your organs. Inflammation is like having a little fire inside you that never quite goes out, and it's implicated in many diseases, such as arthritis, heart disease, and even neurodegenerative conditions. A metabolic reset can help douse those flames, reducing your body's inflammatory response and protecting your health.

Then there's the matter of heart health. An efficient metabolism helps in managing cholesterol levels and reducing blood pressure, effectively taking the strain off your heart and blood vessels. This kind of internal tune-up can make a world of difference in warding off cardiovascular diseases.

But wouldn't you know it, the benefits don't end there. There's this magical process called autophagy, a sort of self-cleaning oven feature your cells possess. During a metabolic reset, particularly when you pair it with certain fasting strategies, autophagy ramps up, clearing out cellular debris and helping prevent diseases like Alzheimer's. It's like giving your cells their very own spa day to rejuvenate and protect themselves.

Let's not underestimate cancer prevention, either. When metabolism is optimized, it means less cellular damage and less oxidative stress—two factors that, if left unchecked, can lead to mutations and cancer. Keeping your metabolism in tip-top shape helps to reduce these risks, keeping your cells healthy and less prone to dangerous changes.

So you see, a metabolic reset isn't just about slipping into a smaller pant size; it's also a profound strategy to extend your lifespan and reduce the risk of many chronic diseases. It's about investing in a body that's not just lighter, but significantly healthier and more resilient for the long haul.

Your metabolism is like the central hub of your body's health network, and by now, it should be crystal clear: taking care of it is non-negotiable. It's not just about the now; it's about a vibrant, robust life for years to come. So, what's next? Read on to learn how to apply these insights to your unique situation and truly transform your health narrative.

Remember, resetting your metabolism does more than rearrange the figures on the scale. It sets you up for a longer, fuller life with reduced risks of debilitating conditions. That's a goal worth striving for, and it's entirely within your reach. Let's step boldly into a world where we not only live longer, but live well.

Conclusion

Your Metabolic Reset Journey

As we come to the close of our exploratory venture into the realm of metabolic reset, it's paramount to reflect on the ground we've traversed together. Comprehending metabolism's complexity, embracing lifestyle adjustments, and fostering enduring health—this odyssey has been nothing short of transformative. Through the lens of scientific insight and practical advice, you've seen how wresting control from a sluggish metabolism can revolutionize your entire being.

Embarking on this journey, you have confronted myths, harnessed the power of nutrition, and discovered the profound impact of intermittent fasting. Detoxifying your body, you've unlocked pathways to metabolic success. You've stepped onto the scales of blood sugar balance and nurtured your gut, knowing that each plays a pivotal role. And let's not forget that without the soothing embrace of sleep or the invigorating rush of exercise, metabolic harmony remains an elusive dream.

Weight loss plateaus—previously frustrating obstacles—are now just part of the process, challenges you're equipped to tackle with determination. Understanding when to supplement your efforts with vitamins, minerals, and adaptogens has added nuance to your metabolic symphony. Meal planning, once a drudge, now dances with creativity and metabolic purpose.

Tracking progress has offered you solid ground in a sea of variable factors, a lighthouse guiding you towards your goals. Every habit you've curated is a brick in the foundation of your healthier self, braced for the ebb and flow of life's irregular tides. Customizing your plan, you've tailored strategies to the unique tapestry of your physiology, environment, and challenges.

Success stories have been lanterns in the dark, inspiring steps forward when doubt loomed. The social battlefield of eating out and the labyrinth of peer pressure are now arenas where you stride with confidence, armed with strategies to preserve the sanctity of your metabolic goals. And in recognizing pitfalls, you've also grown wiser, sidestepping the snares that once might have trapped you unawares.

Your understanding now transcends weight loss—this reset was but the spark of an even vaster expanse of health benefits. Energy spikes that ebb and flow like the tide have smoothed into a steady current. Mental fog has lifted, revealing the sharp contours of clarity. You stand on the cusp of longevity, a future dotted with few preventable diseases and vibrant well-being.

Yet, don't let this conclusion represent a finale. Rather, see it as a commencement, the dawn of your ongoing evolution. Health isn't a static picture but a dynamic panorama, continuously unfurling. Your metabolic journey doesn't end with the last page of this book—it's a narrative you'll keep writing day after day, with each choice serving as a pen stroke in your ongoing story.

Remember, transformation is a process, not a single monumental leap. It's the subtle shifts, the small victories, and the lessons learned from missteps that accumulate into a profound metamorphosis. Patience, coupled with persistence, is the crucible from which your renewed self will emerge—stronger, more vibrant, and in tune with the innate rhythms of your body.

Emerging wiser from this expedition, you know that temptations will present themselves, stress will knock at your doors, and life will throw its curveballs. But you possess now an armory of knowledge, a shield of habits, and the sword of self-efficacy to parry these potential relapses.

In truth, you're not the same person you were at the beginning of this book. Every cell in your body bears witness to the transformation. Your thoughts, radiant with positivity, mirror your physiological rejuvenation. You breathe the air of someone who has not just traversed a path but has widened and smoothed it for others to follow.

As you continue on your path, stay curious. Keep learning and adapting because the frontiers of health and metabolism are constantly expanding. Share your insights, your triumphs, and yes, your struggles too—because every narrative enriches the tapestry of communal wisdom. Others need that light you now carry; share it generously.

Complexities of metabolism notwithstanding, remember the essence of our collective wisdom: listen to your body, nourish it with respect, move with joy, and rest with peace. Each day is a new opportunity to nudge your metabolism in the direction that escalates your vitality. Seize it with both hands!

And so, we part ways at this juncture—not as guide and follower but as fellow travelers on parallel journeys. Yours is a path of continued awakening, mine of ongoing discovery. May the strides we've made together encourage you to embrace a future rich with energy, health, and an unfettered enthusiasm for the vibrance of life.

Your metabolic reset journey doesn't culminate here—it's perpetually unfolding. May you navigate its waters with the resilience of the steadfast voyager, the wisdom of the seasoned captain, and the spark of an undying explorer. Onward, to seas of boundless vigor and horizons of unfathomable health!

About the Author
David Alexander

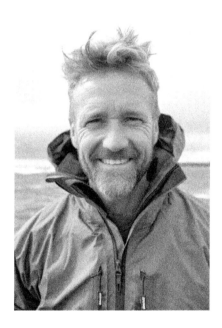

David Alexander is a highly regarded author specializing in weight loss, with a genuine passion for unveiling the truths and myths surrounding diets and weight-loss techniques. With over two decades of extensive research and meticulous study, David is a beacon of reliable knowledge in a field crowded with ever-emerging "fads" and transient trends. He has dedicated his life to discerning what fosters sustainable, healthy weight loss, distinguishing efficacious methods from the ephemeral.

David's journey began 20 years ago when his curiosity led him to delve deep into the myriad diets and weight loss strategies flooding the market. This exploration blossomed into a profound, enduring quest for understanding, positioning David as an erudite in the sphere of weight loss. His comprehensive insight encompasses a broad spectrum of topics, enabling him to dissect and analyze varying approaches to weight loss with exceptional precision and depth.

Married and a proud father of three, David merges his familial experiences with his professional acumen, cultivating an approach that is both profoundly empathetic and exceptionally knowledgeable. His commitment to fostering well-being and health extends beyond the boundaries of his own home, seeking to aid others in navigating their weight loss journeys safely and effectively.

David's mission is clear and unwavering: to guide others toward achieving their weight loss goals through safe, substantiated, and sound methods. He champions the cause of healthy living and strives to illuminate the path for those grappling with weight loss, providing support, knowledge, and encouragement every step of the way.

David's extensive knowledge and commitment to helping others have culminated in a series of weight loss books, designed to empower readers with the tools and insights needed to reclaim their health and well-being. Through his enriching and enlightening works, David Alexander has become a trusted ally for those on their weight loss journey, offering hope and a wellspring of wisdom in a world fraught with weight-loss misconceptions.

One Final Task

Now that you're well on your way to long-lasting, sustainable weight loss and a healthy mindset, you're in the perfect position to hand the baton to the next person. Simply by sharing your honest opinion of this book and a little about your own journey, you'll show new readers where they can finally find the guidance they've been looking for.

IN UNDER 1 MINUTE YOU CAN HELP OTHERS JUST LIKE YOU
BY LEAVING A REVIEW

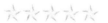

Please use the QR code below to leave your review.

Printed in Great Britain
by Amazon

35581007R00119